INFLUENZA VIRUS

VIRUS

The Inevitable Enemy

INFLUENZA VIRUS
VIRUS
The Inevitable Enemy

George Fu Gao
Chinese Center for Disease Control and Prevention, China
Institute of Microbiology, Chinese Academy of Sciences, China

Alexander Huan Liu
University of Science and Technology of China, China
State Key Laboratory of Virology, China

World Scientific

NEW JERSEY · LONDON · SINGAPORE · BEIJING · SHANGHAI · HONG KONG · TAIPEI · CHENNAI · TOKYO

Published by

World Scientific Publishing Co. Pte. Ltd.

5 Toh Tuck Link, Singapore 596224

USA office: 27 Warren Street, Suite 401-402, Hackensack, NJ 07601

UK office: 57 Shelton Street, Covent Garden, London WC2H 9HE

British Library Cataloguing-in-Publication Data
A catalogue record for this book is available from the British Library.

《流感病毒: 躲也躲不过的敌人》
First published in 2018 by China Science and Technology Press Co., Ltd.

B&R Book Program

INFLUENZA VIRUS
The Inevitable Enemy

ISBN 978-981-125-621-9 (hardcover)
ISBN 978-981-125-622-6 (ebook for institutions)
ISBN 978-981-125-623-3 (ebook for individuals)

For any available supplementary material, please visit
https://www.worldscientific.com/worldscibooks/10.1142/12833#t=suppl

Typeset by Stallion Press
Email: enquiries@stallionpress.com

The first **popular science** book on "Influenza" by Professor George F. Gao, Member of the Chinese Academy of Sciences (CAS), International Member of US National Academy of Sciences (NAS) and National Academy of Medicine (NAM), Foreign Member of Royal Society (London), Member of the German National Academy of Sciences Leopoldina and Director-General of Chinese Center for Disease Control and Prevention, in collaboration with Professor Alexander H. Liu, Prominent Scientist of China Outstanding Science Communication, Ambassador of Health News' Life Hero, Winners of China Excellent Prize of Books for Science Popularization & China Excellent Prize of Videos for Science Popularization, Champion of CAS Challenge for Information Knowledge, Science Popularization Contributor to International Contest for Popular Science Works.

Recommended by

Qide Han, Member of the Chinese Academy of Sciences
Zhu Chen, Member of the Chinese Academy of Sciences
Wei He, Expert of the Chinese Academy of Medical Sciences
Longde Wang, Member of the Chinese Academy of Engineering
Yunde Hou, Member of the Chinese Academy of Engineering
Chen Wang, Member of the Chinese Academy of Engineering
Lanjuan Li, Member of the Chinese Academy of Engineering
Yanhao Xu, Deputy President of China Association for Science and Technology
Zhonghe Zhou, Member of the Chinese Academy of Sciences

Do not hide any more

Let us explore the world of flu viruses
Start our go-with-feel journey of science popularization
50000 Books Sold in 100 Days
POPULAR SCIENCE PRESS

About the Authors

George F. Gao

Dr. Gao is a Member of the Chinese Academy of Sciences, International Member of US National Academy of Sciences, Fellow of The Third World Academy of Sciences, Foreign Member of Royal Society (London), Foreign Fellow of the Royal Society of Edinburgh, and Member of the African Academy of Sciences and Member of the German National Academy of Sciences Leopoldina. He is also the Chief Scientist of the National Science and Technology Major Project for Prevention and Control of Infectious Diseases, Deputy Director of the Ad Hoc Committee on Science Popularization affiliated to the Standing Committee of China Association for Science and Technology, Vice-President of the Beijing Association for Science and Technology, President of the Chinese Society of Biotechnology, Vice-President of the Chinese Medical Association, Dean of the Savaid Medical School, University of Chinese Academy of Sciences, Vice-President of the Beijing Institutes of Life Science, CAS, Director of the CAS Key Laboratory of Pathogen Microbiology and Immunology, Visiting Professor of the University of Oxford, Honorary Professor of the University of Hong Kong, Senior Fellow of the Hong Kong Institute for Advanced Study, Director-General of the Chinese Center for Disease Control and Prevention, and Vice-President of the National Natural Science Foundation of China. He received his Bachelor's degree, Master's degree, and PhD from Shanxi Agricultural University, Beijing Agricultural University, and University of Oxford, respectively, and his postdoctoral training at the University of Calgary, University of Oxford, and Harvard University/Harvard Medical School. He was a lecturer at University of Oxford and the former Director-General of the Institute of Microbiology, CAS. His research interests include interspecies transmission of pathogens, molecular mechanism of infection and host cell immunity, as well as public health policy and global public health strategy. He has published more than 800 refereed scientific papers including *Cell*, *Nature*, *Science*, *The Lancet*, *The New England Journal of Medicine*, etc., and over 10 books. He is the Chief Scientist of the National Program on Key Basic Research Project (973 Project) and a Principal Investigator of NSFC Project for Creative Research Groups. He has been awarded China Youth Science and Technology Award, Tan Jiazhen Grand Achievement Prize and Life Science Innovation Award, Shulan Medical Sciences Award, Wu Jieping–Paul Janssen Medical & Pharmaceutical Awards, National Science and Technology Progress Award, Science and Technology Award-Chinese Medical Association, Science and Technology Award-Chinese Preventive Medicine Association, HLHL Foundation for Scientific and Technological Advancement, HKU Centennial Distinguished Chinese Scholar Scheme, Nikkei Asia Prize, TWAS Medical Science Prize, TWAS Medal Lectures and Russia Gamaleya Medal, etc. He is the author of several professional books, e.g. *Zika Virus and Zika Virus Disease*, and other works.

Alexander H. Liu

Dr. Liu is the Associate Professor of University of Science and Technology of China (USTC), Member of Chinese Society for Microbiology, Board Member of China Science Writers Association, Executive Member of the Beijing Science and Technology Writers Association, Member of Hubei Science Writers Association, and Wuhan Research Association for Science Popularization, Executive Member of Wuhan Intellectual Property Society, Member of Asia-Pacific Biosafety Association, Distinguished Professor of Huazhong University of Science and Technology, former Associate Professor of Chinese Center for Disease Control and Prevention (CDC), former Associate Professor of Wuhan Institute of Virology, Chinese Academy of Sciences (CAS), Expert of the Research Team of the Joint Prevention and Control Mechanism of the State Council against COVID-19, Expert of the Think Tank for "National and Provincial Education Project" Science Classes, Outstanding Science Popularization Contributor in the 70th Anniversary of Science Popularization Work in Hubei Province, and Champion of CAS Challenge for Information Knowledge. He graduated from the State Key Laboratory of Virology, College of Life Sciences (CLS), Wuhan University (WHU), and received his postdoctoral training on medical immunology from the University of Colorado. He was the President of Student Union of CLS, WHU, Vice-President of Graduate Union of WHU, and Vice-President of China Students and Scholars Association of National Jewish Health, USA. His research interests include microbiology, immunology, evolution, as well as biosafety and health education. Professor Liu leads and participates in National Intellectual Property Strategy Project, National Science and Technology Major Project, and National Key Research and Development Project. He has published more than 50 academic and research papers in SCI international or core journals, as well as over 30 popular science articles in *Guang Ming Daily* and other media, such as *Fighting Against HIV: The Protracted Warfare*, and *the Amazing Gene: From the Spider-man to the Hulk*. He was awarded China Excellent Prize of Videos for Science Popularization for two times: *The War Without Smoke of Gunpowder: Humans Versus Flu Viruses*, and *A Go-with-Feel Travel: Interspecies Transmission of Viruses*, the First Prize for CAS Video Competition for Science Popularization for his video works *The Precision-Guided*

Molecular Weapon: Anti-HIV Drugs, and Creative and Excellent Prize for CAS Video Competition for Science Popularization for his video works *Binary Detective: Tracking the Viruses*, and *P4 Iron Man: Wuhan National Biosafety Laboratory*. He has delivered science lectures and classes themed *The Avengers in the Micro-world, Dialectical Thinking and Science Spirit, Are You Ready? An Evolution Adventure!* and *Upgrading Microcosm: Vaccine Saint, Magic Genes- From Spiderman to Hulk* that has reached a 10-million-strong audience, and participated in activities such as Academicians and Experts at School. He has been conferred the honorary titles of Prominent Individual of 2020 China Outstanding Science Communication, 2021 Beijing the Most Beautiful Scientists, An Ambassador of Health News' Life Hero, Science Popularization Contributor to International Contest for Popular Science Works, Outstanding Individual of Hubei Science Popularization in 70 years, Excellent Member of Wuhan Scientists for Science Popularization, etc. He is the author of the book *The Storming of Virus & Human, Life of Peace & War, Little Virus Big World* and the editor-in-chief of *The Pillars of the Biosafety Level Four: National Biosafety Laboratory, Wuhan (P4)*, and other books. His books have been awarded China Excellent Prize of Books for Science Popularization three times, CAS Excellent Popular Science Books, Hubei Excellent Popular Science Books, Beijing Most Popular Books, Wuhan Best 10 Popular Science Books.

About the Translator

Xin Zhang

Ms. Xin Zhang is the International Collaboration and Communications Officer of the Institute of Biophysics (IBP), Chinese Academy of Sciences (CAS). She graduated from Wuhan University and majored in Foreign Linguistics and Applied Linguistics. She was the valedictorian with top GPA from Wuhan University, and has won many awards such as Award of the 13th National FLTRP English Debating Competition, Prize at the 17th English Interpretation Contest of Hubei Province, Prize at the 18th English Translation Contest of Hubei Province, Excellent Student Award, Outstanding Undergraduate Award, Outstanding Postgraduate Award, National Scholarship, etc. She developed proficient language skills required for interpreters and translators when working in academic events and conferences. While working at CAS, she enriched academic activities, created favorable atmosphere for scientific exchanges, and advanced important collaborative relations with overseas counterparts. These efforts achieved stronger representation and helped carry the voice of CAS to the world. She popularized scientific achievements in institute's commemorative events for the 60th anniversary. She served as the interpreter in international conferences, such as the *6th Meeting of Group of High-containment Laboratory Directors*, attended by eight representative countries and Food and Agriculture Organization of the United Nations (FAO); the Opening Ceremony of Wuhan National Bio-safety Level 4 (BSL-4) Laboratory, a symbol of the great success of France–China cooperation; and the MoU signing ceremony for the Sino–Africa Joint Research Center MoU signing ceremony, the first large-scale comprehensive overseas scientific and educational institution built by the Chinese government. She engaged in liaison interpretation for many prestigious scientists, including Nobel Laureates, President of the Royal Society, and French Ambassador to China. She was given credit by CAS in 2016 for high-quality media, ranking No. 2 among over 100 institutes. She was recommended to deliver a keynote speech in the international collaboration and communications training class held by CAS in 2019, and was recognized as IBP Outstanding One twice.

Sculpture: To the Microworld

The sculpture is an artistically designed "opened" influenza virus, suggesting humans will "open" the virion of the influenza virus and conquer it. The virus is split into two parts, rotating up and down. The genomic RNA consisting of eight segments is twisted inside, signifying the close and complex relations between RNA and external characteristics of the virus. Surface proteins are represented by simple cylindrical shapes in different heights, symbolizing the contrast between hemagglutinin and neuraminidase proteins and reflecting the spirit of "pursuing knowledge and achieving ingenuity." The sculpture is located in the Olympic Village campus of CAS.

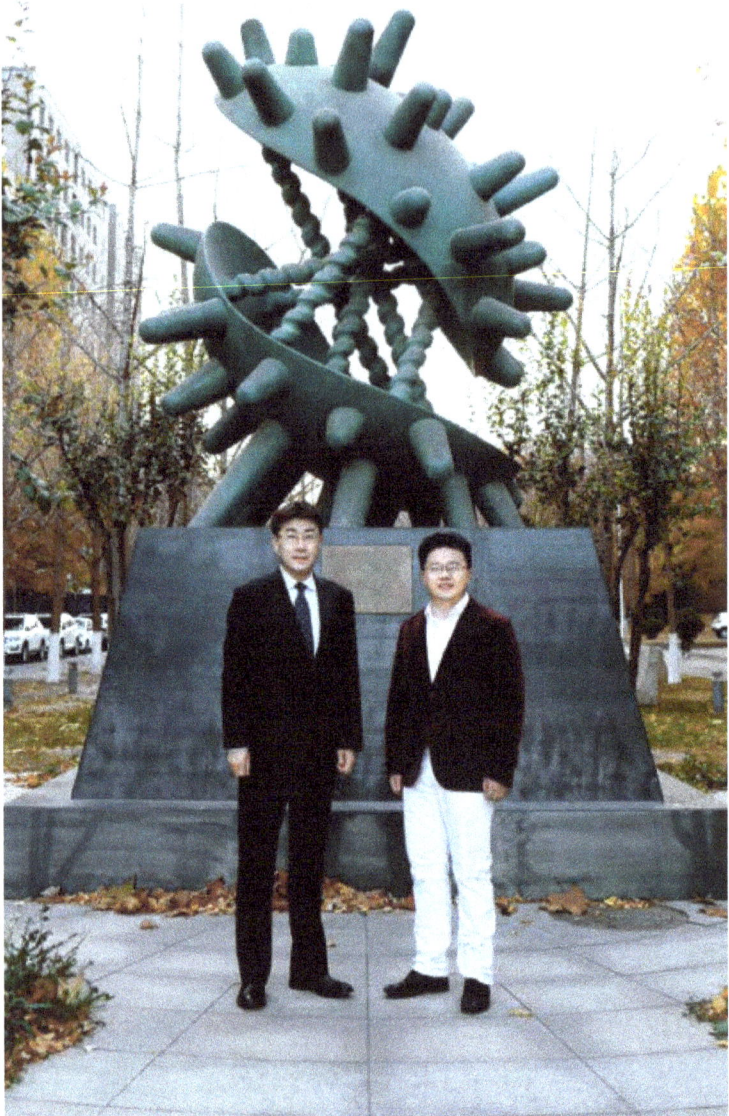

高福（左） 刘欢（右）

Prof. George F. Gao (left) and Prof. Alexander H. Liu (right), in front of the influenza virus sculpture erected in the CAS Olympic Campus, Beijing, China

Preface

The year 2018 marks the 100th anniversary — a centenary — of the global influenza pandemic of 1918!

Today, we have come to know about influenza viruses, which are tiny particles that have been disturbing us for so many years with their frequently mutating forms to confuse us and evade our tracing. All of a sudden, they create waves of disaster in our world.

Now, we are dazzled by the more micro, accurate, and systematic trends with the rapid development of science and technology. The innumerable achievements made in these professional fields, as glistening as blooming fireworks in the night sky, will be preserved in the long river of history and treasury of civilization, with the light of intelligence sparkling like billions of stars.

At least, we have known that flu viruses are just around the corner instead of being far away from us. Nevertheless, with the wish of escaping them, we had thought we could create a living space isolated from flu viruses in a certain spatial state. Therefore, we are always far from ready, either in our actions or in our minds, to fight against the flu viruses.

"Science is by no means a selfish entertainment. Those who are fortunate enough to be devoted to science study, should first and foremost serve humans with their knowledge," said Karl Marx, a philosopher from Germany. To explore natural law is an accumulative process, in which humans should keep forging ahead in unknown fields of knowledge. The gleam of scientific inspiration comes from the discovery of the inherent nature through practice and the abstraction of it into a theory or a trend, rather than the simple establishment of a formula or a model.

According to Louis Pasteur, "Science knows no border, but scientists have their own country." The mission of scientific and technological innovation in the new era is to make achievements in the home soil. Infectious diseases know no national boundaries. Viruses can travel without visas. With the ability of interspecies transmission, flu viruses, free from national and regional restrictions, are ghosts hovering in the Earth's atmosphere.

Only when scientific innovation benefits the public can it be full of vitality, and nothing but the deep-rooted scientific passion in the public's heart can drive continuous scientific and technological innovation. Like the power of spring breeze which can start a great fire with a small spark, science education and communication are capable of popularizing scientific thoughts, knowledge, approaches, achievements, and spirit.

In the universe filled with billions upon billions of stars, viruses follow humans everywhere, just like the Tom-and-Jerry story in the Disney land. There is an alternating circle between life and environment, and mutual enrichment between nature and civilizations. Let us explore flu viruses, the enemies impossible to be avoided, and start our go-with-feel journey of science popularization.

May 28, 2018

Contents

Introduction

As Spring 2018 approaches, the wind remains cool in Northern China as night falls. People jogging or doing sports can be seen from time to time in the runway or avenue of the Olympic Forest Park. Despite a quick glimpse of these figures around the corner, we can still glance at their faces with masks, which seems to reveal the approaching of flu season in a vague way... Time may never stop. The story of the spring shall start with the last season.

Influenza viruses, one of the major viruses on the earth, never says goodbye to humans.

American journalists have produced literary documentary works themed on the Great Influenza in 1918, which have also been translated into Chinese. Many other countries have added influenza knowledge as part of "health" theme to extracurricular readings of children and primary students to help citizens establish the concept of public health. There are many academic and professional works introducing world-class achievements made by both Chinese and world scientists in the field of flu viruses. Some readings on health education are being gradually published in China, disseminating knowledge about public health to more people. The understanding of science by the public can promote the development of the society, and the value of science can serve the public and society.

The profound scientific knowledge concerning influenza will be explained step by step in simple language in 10 chapters this book, from the perspective of influenza history, disease development, immunity and health, life and evolution, society and nation, and world and humans, in such a way that readers will feel like opening a mysterious map to explore the unknown treasure. By telling tales about scientific legends to the potential future scientists, the authors hope to sow scientific seeds in their heart this spring.

Chapter 1, titled Chilly Winter, begins with the story about the sudden invasion of influenza in the winter of 2017. In this chapter, fundamental concepts and terminologies about flu viruses are introduced from the perspective of etiology and epidemiology. Readers will get to know the common sense and general principles of health and disinfection, sanitary measures, and individual protection from the story of the "Four Heavenly Kings" of flu viruses. Then, the "Double Challenges" faced by both patients and doctors, whose concerted efforts are required to protect health, are elucidated from the aspects of pathological development, occurrence of severe symptoms, and clinical manifestations of human physiological diseases. Medical progress is a shared cause pursued by all human beings. With history repeating itself, the infectious diseases shake the fundamental unit of our society, and in particular, threaten national security and the progress of world civilization in a severe outbreak.

Chapter 2, titled World War I, reviews the deadliest influenza pandemic in the recorded history. During World War I, the flu virus availed itself of the great opportunity to widely disseminate when countries involved were busy fighting against each other. For the purpose of controlling and suppressing public opinion, the Great Influenza was dubbed the "Spanish Lady," one of the non-belligerent states, despite its outbreak in belligerent states. However, up to now, people remember more about fierce battles on military frontlines. Only those who suffered from the Great Influenza in person may fully understand the invisible virus caused more devastation than that was caused by the roaring gunfire. People remember and miss their loved ones dying of the Great Influenza, while the true nature of the invisible killer remains unknown. More than ten years have passed, and scientists have made numerous attempts and eventually discovered the flu virus in microbiological assays. However, the tiny images of the flu virus remain to be the fuzzy "Mosaic" for humans.

Chapter 3, titled The Story of the Cows, is a glorious classic example for initiating preventive medicine and defeating viruses. The vaccine technology for "fighting poison with poison" is derived from smallpox, a worldwide infectious disease in the past. According to records, it was our ancestors' significant invention to use the pus of the infected to help others prevent smallpox. There were safety risks of this technology considering its potential toxicity, in spite of its certain preventive effect. Edward Jenner, a British surgeon, opened the door to immunology by finding out the secret of cowpox versus smallpox. On the basis of "Apocalypse" of smallpox vaccine, more and more bacterial and viral vaccines are discovered and developed, and the theoretical framework of cellular and humoral immunity is established in immunology. The three lines of defense in our immune system protect us from pathogens invading. Immunology, the most thriving discipline, contributes to the development of tumor immunotherapy, helping us see the light at the tunnel of curing cancer.

Chapter 4, titled The World of Molecules, ushers a microcosmos for readers to explore life mysteries The invention of electron microscopes, the development of nucleic acid amplification techniques, and the construction of the biosafety laboratories help us protect ourselves by getting close to invisible viruses clearly presented to us, just like enjoying a wonderful voyage in the surging sea. The knowledge about the nature of viruses helps us to know about the vaccines and drugs targeting different viruses. We are now witnessing cutting-edge developments in the emerging field of bio-technology and innovative medical concepts. In this great era, the magic "scissorhand" CRISPR, known as "the Hand of God," presents great potential for gene editing, and CAR-T immunotherapy represents a brighter future for disease treatment in medical fields.

Chapter 5, To Catch a Cold, starts with the common cold in our society. In fact, the cold, a common infectious disease, is originated from the note requesting for leave by the imperial college students in Song Dynasty rather than a medical term. "Gan Feng Bo," means feeling "Feng Xie," or Wind Evil, one of pathogenic factors in the theory of traditional Chinese medicine, attacking our bodies by penetrating the skin and pores. In Qing Dynasty, officials enriched its definition into "Gan Mao," namely one's body apparently influenced by Wind Evil. It remains an excuse frequently used when asking for a sick leave even today. Sometimes, we also name it "Zhao Liang," almost similar to the English expression "Catch Cold." There are similarities between different languages in terms of this certain phrase. "Bacterial cold" is often caused by bacterial infection. The antibiotic developed by humans, effective for fighting bacterial infection, was used widely for treating soldiers infected during World War II. It also serves as a special weapon in fighting bacterial cold. The "Viral Cold" is the viral infection caused by different viruses. In most cases, people infected with such viruses except for flu viruses, can recover with the help of their own immune system to identify and eliminate these viruses, even if there are no effective preventive or therapeutic drugs.

Chapter Six, The Devil, begins with a great outbreak of influenza in Venice, Italy. It was the first time when fearful Italians named the dreaded infectious disease — influenza. All four great influenza pandemics recorded in human history were caused by flu viruses, which wreaked havoc across the globe due to their airborne nature and greater virulence than that of the virus causing common cold. There are different types of influenza viruses. In addition to four "influenza families" we mentioned in Chapter 1, there are many virus subtypes. Particularly, influenza A viruses are further classified into 18 (16+2) hemagglutinin (HA) subtypes and 11 (9+2) neuraminidase (NA) subtypes according to different combinations of HA and NA. It is these various viruses that make people feel swamped in fighting against flu viruses. The key to solving these puzzles is to reveal the nature of influenza virions: a seemingly simple structure with deceptive "sugar bomb," consisting of an inner core of single-stranded viral ribonucleic acid (RNA) and an outer membrane protein for virus infection and release.

Chapter 7, Variation, introduces the "magic weapon" of flu viruses attacking humans. The frequent outbreaks of avian flu in recent years are real examples of variations of flu viruses. In particular, emerging H7N9 and H5N1 influenza virus infections in humans have sounded us the alarm of the urgency to prevent and control influenza. The "interspecies transmission misbehavior" of flu viruses demonstrates one of the distinctive features of RNA viruses, namely, instability of their genetic materials, which determines variations in virus characters. Small variations in influenza virus genes are called antigenic drift, while major changes are called antigenic shift. Humans would suffer from troubles when variations occur in viruses since antigens would possess the receptor binding properties to both avian and human cells. In addition to flu viruses, Ebola virus,

MERS-CoV, Zika virus, and others, jumping from animal hosts to humans, regularly launch waves of fierce attack on humans. Maybe we should also reflect on how to respect "the borders of nature."

Chapter 8, Cause and Effect, elaborates a fundamental principle of "Early Detection, Early Diagnosis, Early Intervention, Early Treatment" in combating flu viruses. Therefore, to give an earlier warning to people, "tracing the virus origin" is needed by setting the goal of discovering natural virus hosts, studying direct origins of infectious diseases, and understanding the balance between man and nature from the perspective of macroecology. There are different cold symptoms and virus variations. Clinical symptoms can serve as one of the proofs to confirm different flu virus infections among the huge crowd, and life elements such as protein, nucleic acid, and live virus of flu viruses should be obtained as on-site proofs for detecting pathogens and diagnosing diseases. Based on clinical symptoms diagnosis and identification of flu virus, different therapies can be adopted, such as symptomatic treatment, antiviral treatment, and treatment for severe symptoms according to specific cases. Meanwhile, necessary health policies and intervene measures should also be adopted as a social norm for virus prevention and treatment as well as public protection to prevent and control the spread of diseases.

Chapter 9, Bidding Game, is a metaphor to decide biannually which flu vaccines should to be designed for frequently changing flu viruses, like multiple-choice questions. All vaccines successfully developed by humans, such as live attenuated vaccines, inactivated vaccines, subunit vaccines, and virus-like particle vaccines, seek a balance between immunogenicity and immunoreactivity in the pursuit of efficacy while ensuring safety. The World Health Organization (WHO) issues the "arrest warrant for flu viruses" every spring and autumn, seasons when people are susceptible to influenza viruses; attaches great importance to three flu viruses potentially attacking people; and predicts and determines which kind of vaccines to be prepared to combat them. Several flu viruses may escape from the global pandemic surveillance network. Is it possible for us to replace the multiple-choice question by single-choice question in preparation for the vaccine exam? The single-choice question is how to develop a universal influenza vaccine, and the answer to that is supposed to be the ultimate goal we should achieve in practice.

Chapter 10, A New Era, is a review of the 1918 Global Great Influenza and the flu virus being one of the causes of emerging and re-emerging infectious disease threats faced by humans in recent years. More unknown viruses will intrude into our society with the rapid globalization and increasingly frequent interactions between men and nature. Drawing lessons from the Great Influenza sweeping across the world a century ago, The Global Virome Project was launched with scientific goals to a better tomorrow for human health. It is no longer a battle or a defense between a single virus and a certain person, but a comprehensive interaction between viruses and the human world as well as their natural affinity across time and space.

It seems that we have innumerable stories concerning influenza for a long time. They come and go, and always appear in disorder. Nearly a century has passed since we discovered flu viruses and began to study them. Reviewing progresses in science and technology, we come all the way to develop constantly the means of disease prevention and control as well as health protection. Then they became some silent past memories but would be awakened time and time again.

The sunshine of science and technology will melt the snow and ice covering the scientific mountain peaks into the spring of science popularization, with the life secrets contained flowing to broad plains, widespread forests, winding mountains, and magnificent cities. The mighty forces of science popularization will nourish and excite the public, who are the deepest roots in the fertile soil of the mountain peaks.

June 20, 2018

Beijing, China

Chapter 1

Chilly Winter

The sudden outbreak of influenza in the winter of 2017 resulted in an abrupt surge in the number of infections. Infected people anxiously waited in hospitals to be treated, and some of them developed severe symptoms, even resulting in casualties. What are the scientific fundamentals for treatment of common cold when it attacks us all of a sudden? For example, what are the mechanisms for using respiratory protection equipment and ensuring relevant disease prevention?

1. Four Heavenly Kings

As the Buddhist mantra goes, "all reality is a phantom, and all phantoms are real." Indeed, life is the hardest mantra to read.

In the new millennium, China is witnessing a period of high influenza incidence, with the number of reported cases in winters of 2017–2018 significantly higher than that of the same period in previous years. Nine diagnosis and treatment measures were particularly formulated in *the Diagnosis and Treatment Plan for the Influenza* to effectively combat the flu pandemic and ensure health and safety of the public.

Dear friends, maybe you are reading this book while waiting to be treated at hospitals. Thus, I will not touch on every topic in detail at the beginning of the chapter. The chapter is designed to help you know such fundamentals of the flu as etiology*, epidemiology, pathogenesis, and pathology, and "strategically tackle the enemy" in your mind with the basic knowledge about the flu.

Etiology

The "Four Heavenly Kings" of flu viruses: A, B, C, D, refer to influenza A, B, C, and D viruses, among which, influenza D viruses are known to infect cattle and pigs, although no human infections have been reported until now. Influenza A viruses are the only influenza viruses known to cause global flu pandemics. Influenza B viruses generally occur locally but can spread widely among humans and cause severe illnesses.

The first human influenza A (H1N1) virus was isolated in 1933. In 1940, Thomas Francis Jr. and T. P. Magill isolated the first influenza B virus from humans. Influenza B viruses are often classified into three main lineages, including the earliest type I represented by strains with B/Lee/40, type II represented by strains with B/Yamagata/16/88 (Yamagata), and type III represented by strains with B/Victoria/2/87 (Victoria).

At present, people are mainly infected by influenza A H1N1 and H3N2 virus subtypes and Yamanaka and Victorian strains of influenza B viruses. According to genetic lineages distance analyzed by molecular evolutionary system, it is predicted that Yamagata and Victoria lineage strains originated in 1969.

Influenza B viruses are often highly specific to the hosts they infect — in addition to humans, seals are also their hosts. Other natural hosts remain to be discovered. Professor Albert Osterhaus, a Dutch scientist, first isolated influenza B virus from an infected harbor seal in 2000 and discovered that the gene sequence of strain B/seal/Netherlands/1/99 was homologous with that of the human influenza B virus that caused an epidemic five years earlier.

Therefore, the origins of influenza B viruses may be traced to harbor seals, the potential natural hosts of influenza B viruses. In addition, people are likely to be re-infected by viruses due to their slow variations in seals under evolutionary pressure.

Unfortunately, the speculation was right. It was the Yamagata lineage strain that caused greater havoc in the 2017 flu pandemic.

Influenza B viruses became the dominant influenza strains around every four years in the earlier years. However, recently, they have become increasingly active worldwide, showing an aggressive momentum of counterattack. During the seasonal influenza surveillance in China, primary strains have also been identified in some regions.

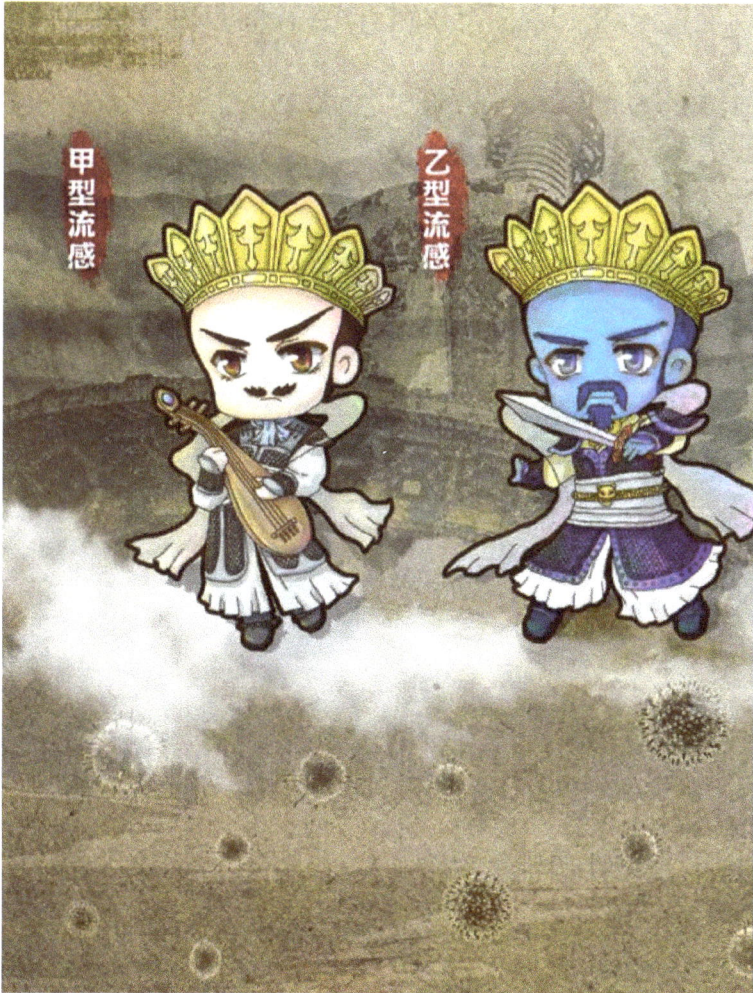

流感 "四大天王"：甲型流感、乙型流感、丙型流感和丁型流感

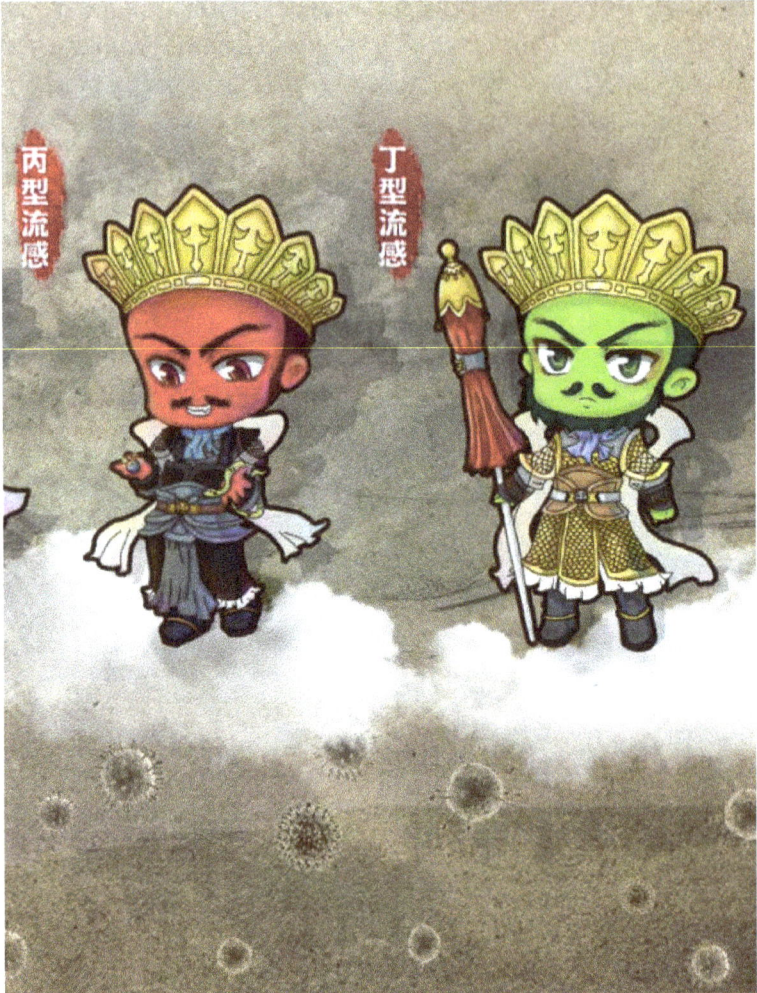

"Four Heavenly Kings" of Flu Virus Families: Influenza A Virus, Influenza B Virus, Influenza C Virus, and Influenza D Virus

Influenza B viruses spread mostly among humans, with clinical symptoms resembling those caused by influenza A viruses such as headache, fever, and muscle ache. In particular, the elderly and children are susceptible to these viruses, which may cause fatal secondary pneumonia and the deadly Reye's Syndrome, leading to organ failure, organ damage, and even death in children.

Most influenza vaccines used at present contain inactivated viruses, with three ingredients (so-called trivalent vaccines): one influenza A (H1N1) virus, one influenza A (H3N2) virus, and one influenza B virus of the same lineage (if there are two different lineages of B viruses in vaccines, they are quadrivalent flu vaccines). Every year, the World Health Organization (WHO) publishes vaccine ingredients to countries worldwide. Victoria and Yamagata viruses have presented different proportions in epidemics around the world since the 1990s. In 2017, we made preparations against Victoria "Fox," only to find it was Yamagata "Wolf" that attacked us.

Sensitive to ethanol, iodine, iodine tincture, and other commonly used disinfectants, as well as ultraviolet and heat, flu viruses can be inactivated in 30 minutes at 56 degree centigrade.

Everyone is an expert on how to disinfect, such as boiling a pot of water to kill the virus, using household disinfectant sprays, wearing super-activated carbon filter masks, etc. However, it should be emphasized again that chemical and physical methods commonly used for eliminating influenza viruses should be supported by scientific evidence.

Take ethanol, iodine, and iodine tincture as examples — the last two are generally finished products, with fixed composition ratio at the time of delivery. For example, iodine is an amorphous combination of elemental iodine (I_2) and polyvinyl pyrrolidone (PVP). Medical iodine, usually low in concentration and light brown in color in 1% or lower concentration, has a broad-spectrum bactericidal efficacy, which can kill bacterial propagators, fungi, protozoa, and other viruses. By the way, the tincture of iodine is also called iodine tincture.

Ethanol, commonly known as alcohol (C_2H_6O), is different from iodine and iodine tincture. Featuring a special, slightly pungent flavor, it can be mixed with water in any proportion. In short, ethanol can be fully mixed into water in any proportion from 0%–100%. However, an ethanol solution with different composition ratios cannot achieve the same disinfection efficacy.

So here is the question: what is the best concentration of ethyl alcohol to kill bacteria?

Ethanol is an organic compound with small molecules featuring great penetration. Its molecules can penetrate from the membranes of bacterial surfaces into the inner cytoplasm, coagulate proteins that are fundamentals of bacterial life, and kill bacteria, the rule of which can also be applied to viral proteins.

Ethyl alcohol is widely used in medical disinfection. While 75% ethyl alcohol is often used for medical disinfection, 95% ethyl alcohol is used for medical equipment disinfection, and 70%–75% ethyl alcohol is used for sterilization. For instance, 75% ethyl alcohol at room temperature (25 degree centigrade) can kill bacteria such as *Escherichia coli* and *Staphylococcus* and other common viruses in a minute.

In general, higher ethanol concentration results in greater protein coagulation. Though ethanol molecules in ethyl alcohol below 70% can enter into bacteria, they cannot completely kill them since they are not "powerful" enough to coagulate bacterial proteins. It was found in a scientific assay that 75% ethyl alcohol can successfully penetrate into bacteria and eliminate bacteria and viruses by coagulating their proteins.

Ethyl alcohol above 95% or even 100% can quickly coagulate protein coatings of bacteria surfaces with its "strong power," contributing to the formation of a "protective wall" for bacteria, which prevents ethanol molecules from getting into bacteria. Thus, bacteria cannot be fully wiped out. Moreover, cells in the bacterial membrane may break through the "wall," revive in right conditions, and wreak continuous havoc on humans.

In terms of their ultraviolet and heat susceptibility, flu viruses can "be inactivated in 30 minutes at 56 degree centigrade." The technique must be familiar to readers majoring or working in the field of microbiology or food industry — indeed, it is the famous "Pasteurization" technique.

In his renowned "broth experiment," Louis Pasteur, a French biologist, proved that there are "bad guys" that cannot be observed directly by our eyes, floating in the air outside the flask with the swan neck. Therefore, the broth and leftovers exposed to the air soon go sour or bad, while the broth in the flask with the swan neck, free from the microbial life, remains fresh for a long time. Of course, we will not debate how Pasteur verified the freshness of the broth at that time.

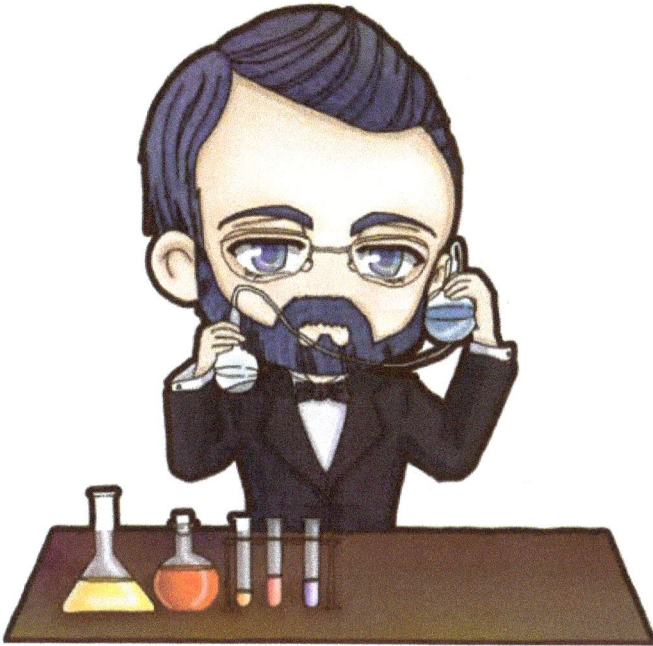

微生物学著名的 "肉汤实验"

The Renowned "Broth Experiment" in Microbiology

Anyway, irrefutable proof from this experiment shows that microbial pathogens have been lurking in the shadows for thousands of years and pose constant threats to our health. Later, a fast and efficient rule was adopted in medical and food industry to eliminate "bad guys": the sterilization punching combination of "56 degree centigrade + 30 min," which can also be used to kill viruses.

Today, we may have a flash of wit while drinking milk: instead of spending half an hour on "braising" the milk at 56 degree centigrade, how about we directly use 100 degree centigrade to sterilize it in three minutes? You may even want to "click the like button" for your brainwave! However, another flash of wit might hit you: does the boiled milk have the same nutrients as before? The effective disinfection procedure will also take away nutrients and "good guys."

Pasteur, the "Patron Saint of Human Health," should be remembered with gratitude for the benefit and wellbeing he brought to us.

Epidemiology

The people who were infected or are in the latent period of infection are the main contagious sources of influenza, either in the late incubation or at acute stages. Infected animals can also spread flu viruses. Limited animal-to-human transmission of flu viruses may occur via close contact. The virus that is mixed in the secretions of its human host can release toxins in the human respiratory tract for three to six days. The period of releasing toxins exceeds one week in human hosts like infants, children, and patients with immune impairment, while it may last one to three weeks for people infected with H5N1/H7N9.

All these mean flu viruses are contagious and can be spread from person to person, people to animals, or animals to people. Thus, they follow general principles for prevention and control of all infectious diseases, i.e., the "three fundamental elements."

The First Step: Source Control

Source control is the most effective way to prevent the spread of infectious diseases. People infected with person-to-person infectious diseases or carrying such disease-causing pathogens should be quarantined appropriately in the designated place in time, temporarily isolated from others, and treated and nursed carefully. Their secretions, excreta, and utensils that may spread the infected viruses should also be disinfected if necessary to prevent the spread of pathogens.

However, it is not easy to identify infectious sources caused by unknown origins or animals since the cause-and-effect inference in epidemiology and sufficient evidence in laboratory assays are hard to be obtained in a short time, particularly in terms of those sudden and acute infectious diseases.

Nevertheless, once the infectious source is identified, it is necessary to adopt efficient measures in time to control it and make sure it will not spread the pathogen to susceptible people. Therefore, it would be wise for anyone infected with influenza

to stay at home and take rest instead of "dragging themselves" to work, so as to benefit themselves and others.

The Second Step: Cut Off the Transmission Path

The most effective way to prevent infectious, insect-borne, and parasitic diseases from spreading through the digestive tract, blood, and other body fluids is by cutting off the transmission path. Primary methods include transmission blocking, sterilizing, and culling. For example, the food or drinking water contaminated with pathogens should be discarded or disinfected; rooms or utensils contaminated should be fully sterilized; used disposable medical supplies should be disinfected or burnt harmlessly; and prevention measures should be adopted during the transmission season of insect-borne infectious diseases.

Meanwhile, it is vital to undertake health education interventions to highly susceptible people. Nowadays, methods of preventing influenza A (H7N9) virus still focus on basic hygiene, frequent handwashing, wearing masks, eating cooked meat, etc. More importantly, refraining from eating live poultry is always stressed and remains to be the most effective way to cut off the transmission path.

The Third Step: Protect Susceptible People

As an important step of preventing infectious diseases, protecting susceptible people is often relatively easier. The best method is to vaccinate them directly against an infectious disease if there is a prophylactic vaccine, such as the infant vaccine schedule, and relevant vaccines for physicians, nurses, and researchers engaged in infectious disease study and treatment, and for poultry industry workers.

The vaccination of susceptible people plays an important role in the prevention and control of infectious diseases, which has been proved by the successful eradication of smallpox with the most effective vaccine in history, continuous drop in hepatitis B infection, and long-term, polio-free condition in China in recent years.

Flu viruses mainly spread via droplets when people are infected with flu cough or sneeze, or transmit directly or indirectly through mucous membranes such as the oral cavity, nasal cavity, and eyes. People may also get the flu by touching an object contaminated with the flu virus. Most human avian influenza infections occur through direct contact with infected animals or contaminated environments.

The scariest thing about flu viruses is that they can travel in the air and are ubiquitous in the natural environment. While we may escape from transmission via blood, other body liquids, skin, and mucous membrane contacts, we cannot cut off their spread through aerosols and droplets since everyone needs air to breathe.

Professional Protective Equipment for Specific Viruses

Masks are anything but "cotton covers." With medical progress, we have recognized for a long time that microbes serve as major culprits of diseases and the adage "disease enters and exits from your mouth" holds true. With progress in material technology, masks are getting more effective and their fit is better. "PM2.5 masks" is a hot word or the "frenemy" of haze in recent years. Does it protect humans from flu transmitted via the air?

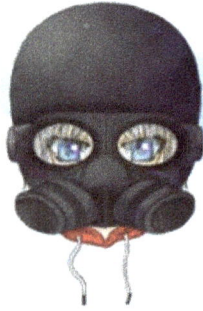
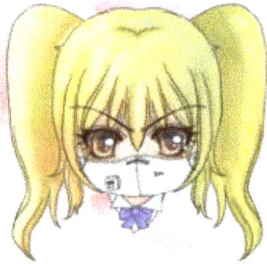

防毒面具   口罩

防护口罩不等于 "防毒面具"

Gas mask   Face mask

Face Mask is Different From Gas Mask

It is Always Good to Wear a Mask

PM, the abbreviation for Particulate Matter, refers to atmospheric particulate matter that has a diameter of less than 2.5 micrometers. PM2.5 masks are manufactured using carbon fiber felt pads and polymer fabric, among other materials. As its name implies, the PM2.5 mask, named based on the air seal that filters molecules of floating particles, refers to the one effective for filtering PM2.5, which means it can successfully filter particles that are 2.5 micrometers in diameter.

What is the size of a flu virus, the biological particle with protruding spikes on the surface? In general, the diameter of a flu virus ranges from 80–120 nanometers. One micrometer is equal to 1000 nanometers, which means a flu virus diameter is less than 0.2 micrometer. Thus, the PM2.5 mask is not enough to filter flu viruses.

However, viruses in the microcosm are not like beans dropping one by one in the macrocosm. "Aerosol" droplets, the major transmission way of flu viruses as we mentioned before, are mixtures "loaded" with virus particles. They can be defined as colloidal dispersion systems consisting of small solid or liquid particles dispersed and suspended in the air or another gas. To put it simply, an aerosol of solid particles is "smoke," and that of liquid particles is "fog."

The Virus is Hiding in the "Smoke" and "Fog"

Viral aerosols are also aerosols, large or small, ranging from 0.01–100 micrometers in diameter. Thus, it seems that certain large and dangerous viruses can be intercepted by PM2.5 masks, which are good for health anyway.

There is another story to share with you:

A young man and a young woman were having dinner together,
"How is the chicken today", she asked.
"Delicious", he said.
She smiled shyly,
and putting a piece of chicken into her mouth.
With an embarrassed smile on her face,
She said, "it seems slightly undercooked".
He said, "everything that you cook is delicious".
They enjoyed a sweet supper together.
...
Consequently, they were infected with avian influenza.

High-temperature cooking!
High-temperature cooking!
High-temperature cooking!
Important things cannot be underscored too much.

We are often afraid of the unknown. With regard to population health, an old Chinese saying comes to mind: "a case involving human life needs to be treated with the utmost care." Several factors affect people's mood, including the psychological and medical diagnosis and treatment for patients in panic, acute symptoms and timely clinical efficacy, the pathogenicity level, and rational drug allocation.

2. Double Challenges

Pathogenesis and Pathology

Influenza A and B viruses initiate infection through binding to surfaces of respiratory epithelial cells containing sialic acid receptors, entering cells via endocytosis, transcribing and replicating virus genomes in the nucleus of infected cells, and producing a large number of progeny virus particles.

These virus particles spread through respiratory mucous membranes and infect other cells. Flu viruses can induce a cytokine storm when humans are infected, leading to systemic inflammation, Acute Respiratory Distress Syndrome (ARDS), shock, and multi-organ failure.

Pathological changes of influenza can be manifested mainly as the tufted exfoliation of ciliated epithelial cells in the respiratory tract, metaplasia of epithelial cells, hyperemia of lamina propria mucosa cells, edema with mononuclear cell infiltration, and others. In severe cases, diffuse alveolar damage may occur.

Diffuse congestion, edema, and necrosis of brain tissues appear in patients with combined encephalopathy.

Inflammatory responses such as myocardial cell swelling, interstitial hemorrhage, lymphocyte infiltration, and necrosis are observed in patients with combined cardiac injury.

It can be concluded from the above passage that flu viruses attack healthy cells in humans, replicate and proliferate new viruses in these cells, and continue to spread and infect other healthy cells. Thus, when the body's immune system is attacked, immune cells will be activated to fight against these viruses and trigger cytokine storms. Organs and their functions will be severely damaged, which may even result in organ failure or death if the inflammatory response is excessive over the human physiological response.

In addition, viruses continue to spread in infected cells and invade human organs such as lungs, brain, and heart. Virus intruders "kidnap" human cells that maintain normal human physiological functions, leading to the damage inside human tissues and organs comprising these cells. By attacking the "defense system," pathogenic bacteria will also take this opportunity to invade and cause mixed viral and bacterial pneumonia with symptoms including lesions, bleeding, and necrosis and result in significant damage or threats to human health and life.

Severe and Critical Cases

Severe flu cases are characterized by one of the following symptoms: persistent fever lasting for more than three days — accompanied by violent cough, pus phlegm, and blood phlegm — or chest pain; fast breathing, difficulty in breathing, and circumoral cyanosis; thought changes: slow to respond, drowsiness, restlessness, convulsions, etc.; severe vomiting, diarrhea, and dehydration; combined pneumonia; or obvious aggravation of pre-existing diseases.

Critical flu cases are characterized by one of the following symptoms: respiratory failure, acute necrotizing encephalopathy, septic shock, multiple organ dysfunction, and other severe clinical conditions requiring intensive care.

Severe and critical illness is related to the fundamental element of human health such as breathing, which is a basic human physiological function. Breathing is the process of gas exchange between the organism and external environment. The human respiratory system mainly works by bringing in oxygen and flushing out carbon dioxide to maintain metabolism. Once an organism stops breathing, its life ends.

The human respiratory system is composed of the respiratory tract and lungs. The respiratory tract, comprising the nasal cavity, pharynx, larynx, trachea, and bronchi, serves as the passage for gas exchange with lungs. Respiratory failure results from ventilation function failure due to various reasons. It leads to inadequate gas exchange and is a clinical syndrome of physiological and metabolic disorders.

If people infected with flu viruses have symptoms of respiratory failure, it means their basic physiological functions are threatened. First aid measures are needed for them to restore the respiratory function while considering viruses or other pathogenic factors. Treating them in a scientific and rational way under existing conditions is a test for both the rescuer and patient, as they face objective and subjective double choices and challenges.

Now we are not going to discuss population and health issues in depth, and we will leave the topic of influenza "for a moment." The Nobel Prize in Physiology or Medicine, a world-renowned prize in natural sciences, will be discussed from the scientific perspective of its establishment purposes and laureates' achievements.

Alfred Bernhard Nobel, a legendary inventor and industry giant, held 355 different patents and set up around 100 companies and factories in 20 countries across the world. In 1895, he set aside his assets worth US$9.2 million to constitute a fund, the annual interest of which was divided into five equal parts to establish five Nobel Prizes, including the one in Physiology or Medicine.

The Nobel Medal in Physiology or Medicine is symbolic of the Genius of Medicine collecting the water pouring out from a rock in order to quench a sick girl's thirst.

There is a Latin inscription inscribed on the medal, literally meaning: it is beneficial to have improved (human) life through discovered arts. The medal is awarded for eminence in physiology or medical science.

Alfred Nobel mentioned two keywords in his last will as for the Nobel Prize in Physiology or Medicine: "discoveries" and "the greatest benefit to humankind." Compared to basic science featuring "discovery" and the clinical science featuring "the greatest benefit to humankind," it seems that the principal guideline of the Nobel Prize is "practice is the sole criterion for testing truth" despite its emphasis on "during the preceding year" as the time requirement. The prize is endowed to those who have

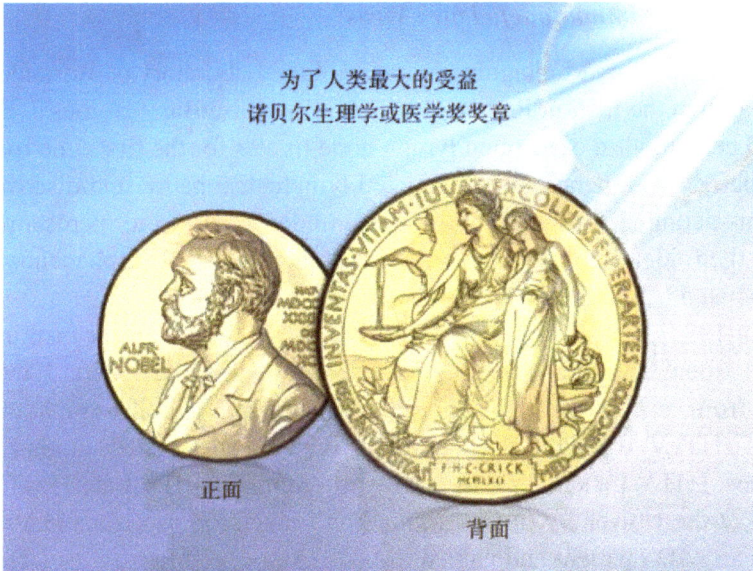

为了人类最大的受益
诺贝尔生理学或医学奖奖章

正面

背面

诺贝尔生理学或医学奖章图案

For the Greatest Benefit to Humankind, the Nobel Medal of Physiology or Medicine (Front and Back). The Images on Nobel Medal for Physiology or Medicine

conferred the greatest benefit to humankind by his or her new but long-tested discoveries widely recognized by the public and applied in medical field.

The Nobel Prize in Physiology or Medicine 2008 was an extraordinary and grand ceremony for virology. It was divided between three European scientists, one half awarded jointly to Françoise Barré-Sinoussi and Luc Montagnier, scientists from the Institut Pasteur for their discovery of Human Immunodeficiency Virus (HIV), and the other half to Harald zur Hausen for his discovery of Human Papilloma Virus (HPV) causing cervical cancer.

By respectively discovering the causes of AIDS and cervical cancer, two deadly human diseases, they have promoted great medical progress and improvement of public health. HIV and HPV, two viruses discovered by the scientists awarded the 2008 Nobel Prize, drew the attention of the public once again.

HIV: Human Immunodeficiency Virus

In 1983, Prof. Luc Montagnier, Director of the Laboratory of Tumor Virus Research in the Institut Pasteur, and Prof. Françoise Barré-Sinoussi, cultivated cells in vitro of swollen lymph node tissues for the first time from a gay person with persistent generalized lymphadenopathy, and discovered a virus acting as a reverse transcriptase under an electron microscope. It was then identified as a novel virus and named Lymphadenopathy Associated Virus (LAV).

In 1984, Prof. Robert C. Gallo, from the National Cancer Institute at the National Institute of Health, isolated a novel virus peripheral lymphocyte from an AIDS patient and called it Human T Cell Lymphotropic Virus (HTLV III), before which, Prof. Gallo had isolated another two viruses, HTLV I and HTLV II, totally different from HIV. Later, Prof. Jay Levy at the University of California, San Francisco, also isolated a virus from an AIDS patient and named it AIDS-Associated Retrovirus (ARV).

In June 1986, the International Association of Microbiological Societies and International Committee on Taxonomy of Viruses used the official name HIV to refer to the three viruses above, due to their complete consistency in morphology, nucleic acid sequence, protein structure, cell tropism, etc.

By mainly attacking helper T cells of the human immune system, HIVs integrate themselves with the host cells permanently and are hence impossible to be eliminated. HIV is a modern "Trojan horse" virus, damaging the human immune system and forcing patients to lose their immunity and resulting in failure to protect themselves from various diseases.

Since its discovery, humans have been fighting hard against this infectious disease.

HPV: Human Papilloma Virus

The HPV particle was discovered for the first time under an electron microscopy in 1949. It is a spherical and symmetrical polyhedron of 20 faces, and 45–55 nanometers in diameter, which is one-thousandth of that of the human hair.

HPV causes infections of the skin and mucous membranes. To date, about 170 different types of HPVs have been fully identified. Some HPV infections are manifested by warts and even cancer, while the majority of the people infected with HPV have no clinical symptoms. "Mild" and weird, HPV does not aim to kill cells as HIV or HBV does.

According to their pathogenicity, HPV can be divided into "high-risk" and "low-risk" types based on their different carcinogenic abilities. Fifteen high-risk HPV types cause cervical intraepithelial neoplasia and cervical cancer. HPV 16 and HPV 18, discovered by Prof. Hausen, belong to high-risk HPV types.

Prof. Hausen's team successfully cloned HPV 16 from cervical cancer specimens in 1977, gradually unveiling mysteries of cervical cancer: HPV 16 was identified in half of cervical cancer specimens and the later-discovered HPV 18 was found in 17%–20% of cervical cancer specimens. An increasing number of results supported Prof. Hausen's conclusion. In 1991, a large-scale survey on epidemiology confirmed that HPV was indeed the "culprit" of cervical cancer.

According to the 2008 press release of the Nobel Committee, Harald zur Hausen went against the current dogma. His discovery led to an understanding of the relationship between HPV and cervical cancer and the development of prophylactic vaccines against HPV acquisition.

Clinically, HIV and HPV are chronic viruses with persistent infection symptoms and can cause severe diseases — AIDS and cervical cancer, respectively — both of which are the ultimate destroyers of human health. However, prophylactic vaccines against HPV can be developed to prevent cervical cancer, although with the same science principles, we are still unable to develop HIV vaccines to prevent AIDS.

We will not elaborate virology and immunology theories, differences between these two viruses, and their disparate host tropism in human cells, but will present a fact to you:

> If HPV had not been identified as the cause of cervical cancer, it would be impossible to successfully develop HPV vaccines;
> Even if HIV has been recognized as the cause of AIDS, it doesn't necessarily mean successful development of HIV vaccines.

With its inherent laws, science is always a road full of dangers and obstacles with the unknown darkness or higher peaks ahead. Instead of building a majestic and magnificent palace for science on the basis of existing theories, we need more courage and faith to move on after numerous failures in the exploration of the origin of life.

Maybe this is the essence of the water image inscribed on the Nobel Medal of Physiology or Medicine. There is no end to exploring the mysteries concerning health. Looking back, on their quest to be healthy, humans have conquered diseases one after another with their blood and tears. Looking forward, confusion and obstacles remain on the human journey toward good health.

The first three Nobel Prizes were established in Physics, Chemistry, and Physiology or Medicine. If basic research serves as the "source" of scientific development, the source is supposed to be all natural sciences. In addition to basic research, research in physiology and medicine is also committed to the greatest benefit to humankind, namely, clinical research.

Adhering to the principle of "focusing more on clinical effects rather than experimental mice," Prof. Hausen discovered HPV, which causes cervical cancer. Irrespective of the interdisciplinary medical study or technological innovation, medical research should focus on medical problems.

The treatment of a single patient is a health question, of 100 patients is a social problem, and of 10,000 or more patients may become a safety issue. Outbreaks of major diseases in history often led to public health crises, which in turn exerted negative influences on national security. The Antonine Plague in Roman Empire was a classic example.

3. The Triumph of Death

The epic historical action-drama film, *Gladiator*, has gained global popularity since it was released in the year 2000. Maximus, a prestigious Roman general with great achievements in battles, is appreciated and cultivated by the Roman Emperor, who wishes Maximus to succeed him as regent to rule the Roman Empire. However, Commodus, the emperor's son, murders his father and seizes the throne. The new emperor proceeds to arrest and kill Maximus and his family. Although he escapes death, Maximus is reduced to slavery and trained to be a gladiator. He searches for opportunities to approach Commodus to avenge the murder of his family and his emperor, thus lighting the fuse of the fall of Roman Empire.

The historical film is a magnificent epic of war and peace, betrayal and faith, and hatred and love in the late Roman Empire seen through the human struggle on and off the battlefield. Faced with the rise and fall of the Empire and ups and downs of his own fate, the gladiator sighs with emotion:

"Death smiles at us all. All a man can do is smile back."

Deeply moved by the movie, we cannot help wanting for the downfall of the emperor. Let us move away from our emotional waves and return to the rational reality: the full name of emperor was Marcus Aurelius Antoninus Augustus, a renowned "emperor philosopher" in the history, who was also the author of *The Meditations* (*Τὰ εἰς ἑαυτόν*) and the last emperor of the Golden Age of the Roman Empire.

More surprisingly, the famous "Antonine Plague" in human history was named after Marcus Aurelius Antoninus Augustus, the emperor endowed with both civil and martial virtues. He was not only an outstanding political leader, but also an extraordinary military commander. During his reign of the Roman Empire (161–180 C.E.), troops returning from wars in the Near East brought in the deadly infectious disease to Roman Empire.

The plague lasted from 164–180 C.E., almost the entire reign of Marcus Aurelius Antoninus Augustus. Lucius Verus, who was the co-emperor along with Marcus Aurelius Antoninus Augustus, died from the plague in 169 C.E., and Marcus Aurelius died 11 years later from the same illness. This natural disaster swept through the entire Empire.

The Roman historian Dio Cassius estimated 2,000 deaths per day in Rome at the height of outbreak, accounting for one-fourth of the infected people. In total, about five million people were killed. A third of the entire population perished in some areas, greatly weakening the Roman Empire.

There are also shocking descriptions by Roman historians about the several plague outbreaks of the Empire.

"Sometimes, when people are chatting while looking at each other, they start to shake and then fall on the street or at homes. When a person is making his handcrafts with a tool in his hand while sitting there, he may also fall aside and have an out-of-the-body experience."

"In the mist of the sea, there are ships with their crews attacked by the wrath of God turned into tombs floating on waves."

"All people in every might city, region, territory, and kingdom, are played by the plague like a ukulele."

The Roman Empire, which originated from the Italian peninsula, eventually grew into vast empire spanning Europe, Asia, and Africa after hundreds of years of territorial expansion through numerous wars of conquest. It began to decline irrevocably in the 3rd century after the outbreak of a series of crises. A series of great plagues spreading since the 2nd century represented a starting point for the fall of Roman Empire from another perspective.

Great political, economic, and cultural achievements were made at the height of the Roman Empire, which could only be rivaled by the Han Dynasty of China in the east at that time. There is always a similar turning point in history. In the late 2nd century C.E., the once-mighty Empire suddenly fell into a decline. Meanwhile, the Han Dynasty in the oriental world was replaced by the Three Kingdoms period.

The late Eastern Han Dynasty refers to the period from the first year of Ping in the Han Dynasty to the 25th year of Jian'an (184 to 220 A.D.), when many heroes and talented rulers fought for territories and power of the central government. The wars led to massive loss of civilians, which was worsened by the following plague. The sudden outbreak of "typhoid" pandemic killed many people from 204 A.D. to 219 A.D.

At the Seaside-Beidaihe (to the tune of Lang Tao Sha)
By Mao Zedong
"Nearly two thousand years ago ,
Wielding his whip, the Emperor Wu of Wei, rode eastward to Chiehshih;
His poems survive."

Cao Cao, the Emperor Wu of Wei, was the hero in chaos at that time. Though he had the aspiration to control the Han Emperor and command nobles and the wiliness to boast command of 800,000 troops in the Battle of Red Cliffs, he also showed his sorrow and sympathy for those suffered in wars and plagues, which could be found in his poem To the Tune of Haoli Xing,

> "While armour lies bloody and wormy.
> Wars raging, people are dying.
> Ungathered bones strew the wilderness---
> for thousands of miles, not a rooster to be heard---
> One tenth of the populations may have ever survived.
> What a heartbreaking disaster!"

According to ancient official records, the total population before the plague outbreak was 56.5 million in the third year of Yongshou period (157 A.D.) of Emperor Huan of Han. However, only 120 years later, in the first year of Taikang period (280 A.D.) of Emperor Wu of Jin, the total population was reduced by three quarters to around 1.6 million in the aftermath of the sweeping plague.

By the end of the Three Kingdoms period, the population of the Central Plain, the epicenter of the plague, was only one-tenth of that in the Han Dynasty. Though the wars and famine at that time played an important role in population decline, the loss caused by the plague was also substantial. Zhang Zhongjing, the famous physician during later years of the Eastern Han Dynasty and the Sage of traditional Chinese medicine, witnessed the great plague.

In the *Original Preface of Treatise on Cold Damage Disorders and the Miscellaneous Illness*, he wrote:

> "My clan was originally many in number, numbering in the area of more than two hundred people. Since the Jian'an reign period (196–220), it has not been ten years, and yet those who have died represent two-thirds. Of those, the number stricken from cold damage amount to seven out of ten. Moved by those who have withered to death in the past and pained by those who could not be rescued from their ultimately deaths...All these have been used to make the Treatise on Cold Damage Disorders and the Miscellaneous Illness, a text that altogether amounts to sixteen rolls. Although the resultant work cannot cure all illnesses, it can

probably be used to apprehend the illness and understand its cause. If one is able to use what I have collected, then they will know more than most."

During the Jian'an reign period, while practicing medicine throughout the country, he witnessed the damages caused by various epidemics on the people.. He summed up his medical experience and study on typhoid fever with decades of painstaking efforts to finish his *Treatise on Cold Damage Disorders and the Miscellaneous Illness,* the first medical work in China on the diagnosis and treatment of diseases. Typhoid fever is a general term for diseases caused by exogenous bacteria including plague.

After wars in the Three Kingdoms period, the unified Western Jin Dynasty was established. However, the Disaster of Yongjia (311 C.E.) led to the Uprising of the Five Barbarians, throwing northern China into disorder, which lasted 130 years. Eventually, the seemingly mighty central dynasty, reluctantly confined to a certain area, gradually fell into decline due to the population reduced by the plague in Eastern Han Dynasty and a series of civil wars of the Sima clan in the Western Jin Dynasty.

We cannot help but wonder why these two once-powerful empires with splendid civilizations that had far-reaching influence weakened and eventually ended.

Reading the ancient official records to review the age of turbulence, we may also find:

The Marquess of Champion Worshipping God of Khentii Mountains to Commemorate the Victory
In the sixth year of Yuanshou (117 B.C.), Huo Qubing, the young Cavalry General of Han Dynasty and the Marquess of Champion, with his heroic dreams vanishing in Jiuquan County, died from an infectious disease. Emperor Wu of Han Dynasty awarded Huo a jar of precious wine for his achievement in leading troops into the Western Regions to defeat and chase the Huns out of Yumen Guan. Huo poured the wine into a creek to share it with all his soldiers. However, the upstream of the creek, which would pass by the Han soldiers had been "poisoned" by enemies with the cattle and sheep plague through the curse of the Huns. Unfortunately, Huo Qubing, the famous general, was infected and eventually killed by the invisible plague.

The Malicious Catapult

In 1346 A.D., the Tartars laid siege to Caffa, Genoa, resulting in a year-long deadlock between the two sides. The Tartars catapulted plague-infested corpses into the town in an effort to infect their enemy. Plague and death soon spread throughout Caffa, resulting in the death of the defenders without fighting and the occupiers abandoning the city at last. All ports of Eastern Roman Empire refused the disembarking of Caffa disaster survivors, and their ships arriving in Venice, Italy, were required to be quarantined for 40 days in the sea before landing. However, beyond everyone's expectations, germ-carrying rats on the ship could swim to the shore. Thus, the horrible Black Death began to spread Europe. The Black Death, which ravaged Europe between 1347 and 1351, killed 25 million people, estimated to be one-third of the total European population at that time, and almost destroyed the European civilization.

What is the truth of the human history that we are reflecting on?

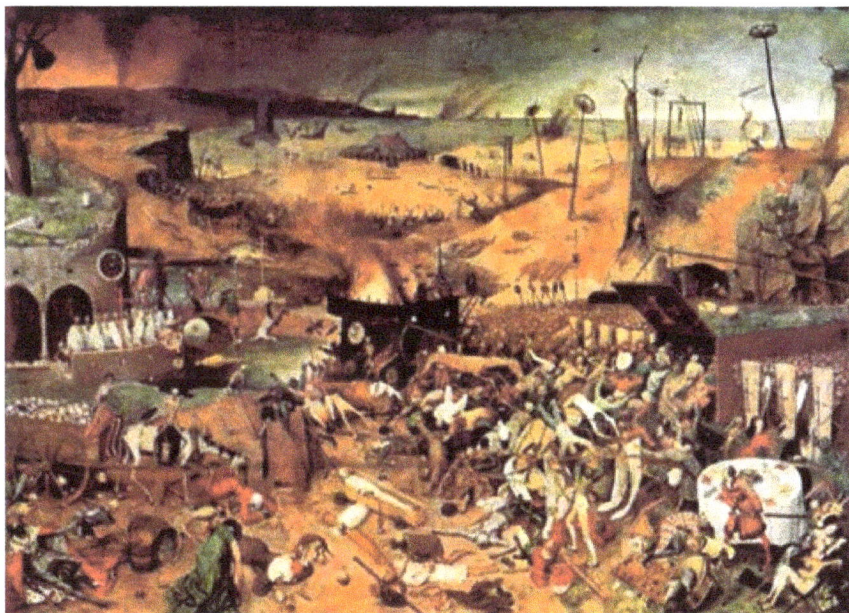

油画《死亡的胜利》：中世纪欧洲的 "黑死病"

Oil Painting: *The Triumph of Death*: "The Black Death" in Mid-Century Europe

Chapter 2

World War I

Human life seemed so fragile in the "meat grinder" battlefields of Verdun and Somme amidst the flames of World War I. However, there was a more brutal and horrible battle waiting, against "death," without gunfire on the rear.

1. "Spanish Lady"

The year 1918 marks the end of World War I and the reshuffling of the global hegemony and imperialism. For the Chinese, we were more impressed by Comrade Li Dazhao's article published in *New Youth,* "The tocsin of humanism has sounded. The dawn of freedom has arrived. The future world is the world of red flags!"

The First World War, or World War I, was an all-out war for global hegemony, in which global colonies and semi-colonies were almost carved up by imperial powers. There were around 30 belligerent nations involved in the four years of World War I, including the German Empire, the Austro-Hungarian Empire, the Ottoman Empire, the Kingdom of Bulgaria, Great Britain, the French Third Republic, the Russian Empire, the Kingdom of Italy, and the United States of America. One and a half billion people were involved in this war, with some 10 million people dying and 20 million wounded.

Together with guns and artillery, tanks, known as a kind of ground warfare, found application in World War I. Airplanes were also put to use to defend airspace during the war. Moreover, some new gas weapons were developed in World War I. The weather forecast served as an important intelligence tool in the war: poison gas could only be "fired" to the battlefield of the enemy using the wind. Therefore, no matter who used the poison gas, the result would depend on the wind direction, with the "muzzle" determining life or death. As the Chinese saying goes, "either the west wind prevails over the east wind or vice versa."

When a yellow cloud drifted over the battlefield, upon hearing their coughing and sneezing from trenches, experienced commanders required their soldiers to wear gas masks. When the battle was finally over, survivors from the frontline complained to other soldiers about their bad luck on the day they felt dizzy and drowsy due to the gunfire.

Several days passed since the gas war. However, soldiers continued coughing. Moreover, more people showed similar symptoms, and there were even severe infected cases. Military doctors, with the horrible term "plague" hovering in their minds, started to doubt their diagnosis about this gas sequela. However, the situation became more urgent.

On March 4, 1918, a person from Haskell County, Kansas, who was infected with severe influenza, was enrolled for military service in Camp Funston. Unsurprisingly, within three weeks, 1100 soldiers at Camp Funston were seriously infected and admitted to the hospital. In the spring of 1918, the flu ravaged 24 of the 36 largest army camps. Furthermore, 30 of the 55 largest cities in the United States — most of them close to military bases with infected soldiers — suffered from the dreaded April.

General Erich von Ludendorff, Commander of the German Army wrote, "It was a grievous business having to listen every morning to chiefs of staffs' recital of the number of influenza cases, and their complaints about the weakness of troops." Despite Spanish neutrality during World War I, Alfonso XIII, the King of Spain, became gravely ill with the flu, an innocent bystander caught in the crossfire.

The flu did not spread widely in Spain until May. However, Spain was neutral and thus under no wartime censorship restrictions on reporting diseases and other news that may damage morale during wartime. Thus, the flu outbreak "leaked out" from the Iberian Peninsula. What's worse, it was widely reported to the world that the King of Spain was severely infected with the flu. The flu was then dubbed "the Spanish Flu" or the gentle killer "Spanish Lady."

Next, the flu spread to Portugal, the country sharing a border with Spain, then to Greece. In June, the flu appeared and quickly spread in Germany. By June and July, it spread to Britain, as well as to colder and regions farther away such as Denmark and Norway, with the death toll rising day by day.

The flu symptoms were recorded in a U.S. military report, "Fulminant pneumonia and lung congestion" and "death within 24–48 hours of illness onset," which were greatly different from those of the common pneumonia. The death rate of the flu was high, and even more unusual, in Louisville, Kentucky, 40% of the deaths occurred in the 20–35 age bracket. All signs pointed to "a new disease."

Eight million Spaniards were infected with the flu during this period. However, they called it the "French Flu" rather than the "Spanish Flu."

Nearly 700 people with severe symptoms from a small (1000 people) military post in France were admitted to hospitals in May, among whom 49 died from the flu infection. General Erich von Ludendorff was not the only commander worrying about the situation. Among two million British soldiers in France, 1.2 million were "attacked" by the flu from June to August. Little was known about the military actions that would be adopted by the German Generals if they had got this news at that time. Maybe they would have no choice but to discuss it at the sand table at the end of the year when the war had ended. Moreover, this was just the first wave of the pandemic.

The "Spanish Lady" killed 40 million people in 1918. Over 100 million deaths were estimated due to this catastrophe worldwide, half of which were young people of a marriageable or childbearing age. Thus, it was called "double death" at that time. More frighteningly, nobody knew the "Black Hand" behind this disaster.

2. The Story of Philadelphia

Misfortunes never come alone. People were still unaware of the death's shadow hanging over Philadelphia and the clouds of World War I.

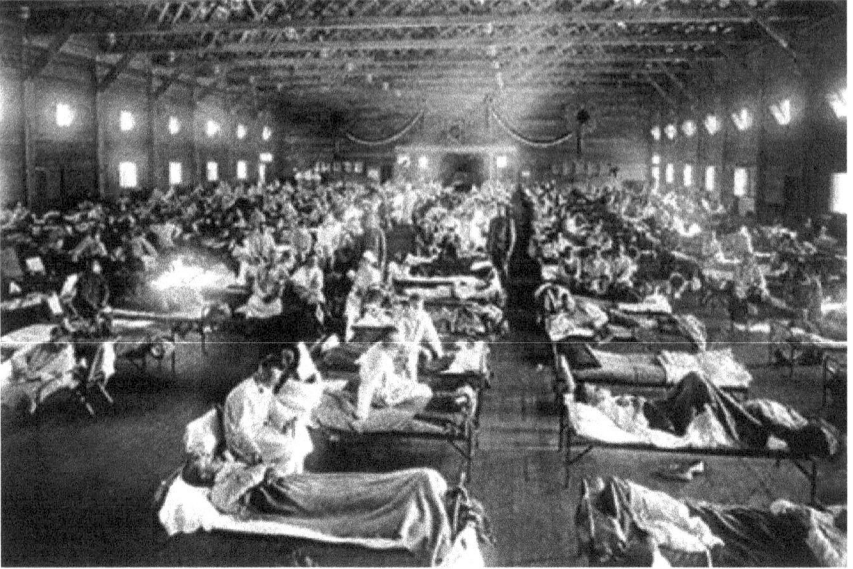

"1918大流感" 治疗营房

The Treatment Barracks for Infected Patients for the "1918 Pandemic"

On September 7, three hundred sailors from Boston arrived at the Navy Yard in Philadelphia. As the birthplace of America's industrialization, Philadelphia had a large population of 1.75 million then, where four extended families were crowded into an apartment with two or three bedrooms, sharing beds as if the members worked in shifts, and their children were even "stacked up" side by side.

Within four days of their arrival in Philadelphia, 19 of these men reported flu symptoms. Despite the remedial quarantine measures adopted, the flu sneaked into the bay. One day later, another 87 soldiers were infected and hospitalized. Three days later, 600 more people became seriously infected with the flu. Then, there was a surge in the number of infected people every minute.

The decisive moments of World War I approached. The United States began to fully activate its war machine. Two million American troops were on their way to invade France and another two million would also be sent there. The war would be expanded, troops would be mobilized, and morale would be boosted. On September 28, hundreds of thousands of people gathered for the three-kilometer parade for war mobilization. Philadelphia, always full of people, created a wonderful "banquet" welcoming the "Spanish Lady".

Two days later, a statement, like a prophecy, was issued by the government reporting similar flu cases among civilians as those in the army.

Military training in the barracks was completely canceled. The flu had taken the lives of these junior soldiers even before they had participated in the war, having neither been sent to the European battlefields nor even meeting their enemies.

On the third day, there were no empty beds for infected people in 31 hospitals in Philadelphia. On the fifth day, all public places were closed and all gatherings were banned. "The flu has peaked" and people woke up the next day only to hear of one flu case after another.

"The door to almost every other house in the Spring Garden Street was covered with the silk, which meant someone's death in this family."

"My uncle was dead... my aunt survived him, and their son was only 13 years old...many newly married young people died first."

"Coffins were piled up outside funeral homes...people started to steal these coffins...their behavior in fact was similar to grave robbery."

The rumor of the return of the Black Death spread like mist among the crowd. The entire Atlantic, Gulf of Mexico, Pacific, and Great Lakes regions were attacked by the flu without exception. Twenty percent flu patients at hospitals in Philadelphia were found dead the next morning by the medical staff. Newly hospitalized patients lying in beds were unable to understand why others looked so helpless.

People were not only frightened by the disease but also by the "fault lines" it created in the family, since the primary targets were the strong young men.

According to the data classified by different age groups in the United States, the largest number of deaths were among those aged 25–29, followed by those aged 30–34, and then 20–24, which was an extremely rare and unusual disease phenomenon. The death toll of those aged 20–40 in Chicago was as five times that of those aged 41–60. In South African cities, 60% of those who died were aged 20–40. A Swiss physician said he had not seen anyone infected over the age of 50 with severe symptoms. France termed this phenomenon as "double death at an early age."

Death from the flu peaked again during the week of October 16. 4600 people were directly killed by the flu or pneumonia. "Even if there was a war, it just passed by our side...but now the fatal disease is standing at the door." "I'm afraid to talk to others, it's like saying 'Don't breathe on me'," recalled someone from Philadelphia. "I was required to put the money on the table. Only after the disinfectant was sprayed all over was it picked up," states a message written by someone from Massachusetts. Ten percent of the total population of Chiapas, Mexico, was killed by the flu.

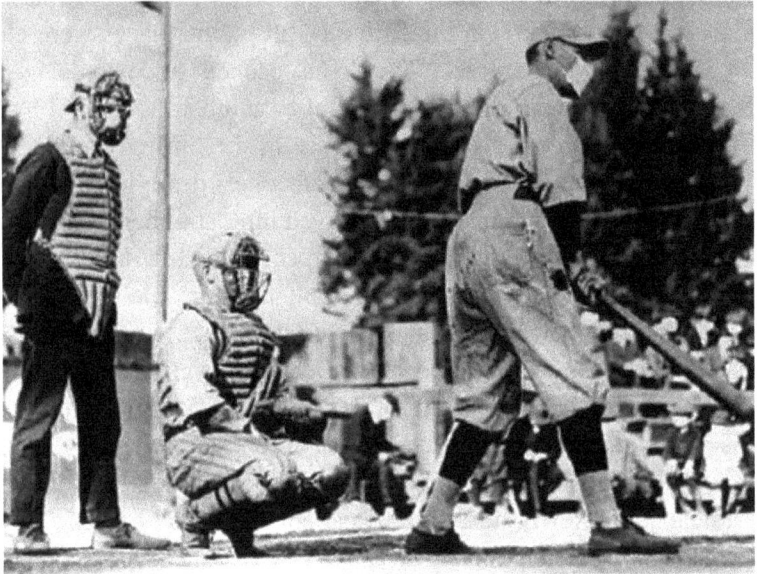

1918 年，棒球比赛运动员戴着口罩参加比赛

In 1918, Baseball Players Wore Masks During the Game

The death rate was 7% in Russia and Iran.

Twenty-two percent of the total population of Samoa in the South Pacific died from the flu.

The mortality rate among those hospitalized for the flu reached 27.3% in Frankfurt, Germany.

Half of the population was infected with the flu in Chongqing, China, and over one-third of the population in Japan.

It is estimated that more than 20 million people were infected with the flu across the Indian subcontinent. The actual numbers may be higher.

At least one-third of the population passed away due to the flu in the Arctic Labrador.

The whole world was affected by this health crisis. There was evidence of the flu infecting people everywhere in the world.

According to a survey by the American Medical Association in 1927, around 21 million people were killed by the Great Influenza pandemic worldwide. According to estimation by scientists in the 1940s, the death toll was between 50 million and 100 million. Data analysis in 2002 revealed 50 million deaths. Behind these figures, the mortality rate was the highest among those aged 21–30.

The flu began its aggressive attack in 1918 during the winter when people were in misery. In December, the dreaded plague seemed to start its second wave. Bad news about the flu outbreak in regions continued to aggravate people's fragile nerves: There were 1700 infected cases reported in St. Louis within three days; the second wave of flu spread in Charleston; the exacerbated flu spread wide in Phoenix; and San Francisco was severely attacked by the flu.

Endowed with its natural geographical barrier of the Pacific Ocean, Australia implemented strict quarantine measures for boats arriving at its port to prevent the entry of the virus to the continent. However, when soldiers from European battlefields returned to Australia by the end of the war, Australian people were really scared of the aggressive flu they brought with them.

In 1919, the flu began to gradually change from a widespread attack to a targeted attack on certain areas, despite some sporadic attacks around the world. Another 11,000 people died from the flu in Chicago in the first two months of the following year. Then, to everyone's surprise, the flu silently retreated and disappeared after 1920.

The Treaty of Versailles was signed by the Allied victors and defeated Central Powers at the end of World War I. "This is not peace. It is an armistice for 20 years", said Ferdinand Foch, the Supreme Allied Commander.

The death toll in World War I was far less than that of the Great Influenza. Where was the foe?

The flu virus was not discovered and identified as the culprit until many years later after people had cast away the shadow of death. The virus, a "substance" between the living and non-living, was discovered for the first time in the tobacco leaf, using a "filtering" method to obtain its nanometer "particle" image under an electron microscope. The truth was finally revealed.

3. Contagium Vivum Fluidum

Since the first day of the disease outbreak, all scientists had worked feverishly round the clock in the laboratory. Every scientist was full of hope and increasingly felt his lack of knowledge about the world when he desperately tried to explore the unknown. "Doctors today know no more about the flu than those did about the Black Death in 14th-century Florence."

The flu was the focus of the medical community in the 1920s. At first, a certain kind of haemophilus influenzae was considered to be its pathogenic bacterium, such as Yersinia pestis, discovered by Alexandre Yersin in 1894, responsible for causing the plague (Black Death). In 1928, Alexander Fleming observed the bacterial-killing effects of penicillin in his study on staphylococcus aureus, but it had no effect on haemophilus influenzae.

It was also thought that the flu pathogen was a bacterium. Among microbes discovered at that time, "It has the best claim to serious consideration as the primary etiologic agent, and its only competition is an unidentified filterable virus." In 1931, Richard Shope, an American scientist, first isolated the influenza A virus from infected pigs and published his findings about swine flu in the *Journal of Experimental Medicine*. His findings were followed by his colleagues isolating the influenza A virus from humans. Therefore, he put forward that "the virus causing human flu is actually the same one causing swine flu." However, it was not until 1933 that the first human flu virus was isolated by British scientists and named H1N1. From then on, influenza was known to be caused by the flu virus. In 1943, the flu virus was finally identified under an electron microscope.

Thus, it took more than 20 years to find out what was responsible for the flu: It was a historical truth that there was no truce.

The gradual establishment of microbiology and bacteriology by Pasteur, Koch, and other scientists opened the door to the microbial world for humans. Enthusiastically searching for bacteria lurking around the corner, humans believed it was only a matter of time before we could grab our disease-causing foes by the throat. However, without taking viruses that were smaller than bacteria into consideration, humans seemed to leave no room for exploring microbes.

After his discovery of the New World, Christopher Columbus returned to Europe with a new species of plant — tobacco, a current global industry, which quickly became prevalent among smokers at that time. With tobacco being planted worldwide, a problem gradually came into being: tobacco mosaic disease.

In 1883, Adolf Eduard Mayer, a German scientist, discovered that the sap from affected tobacco leaves could infect healthy ones. Without discovering the pathogenic microorganism in the sap, he believed that the tobacco mosaic disease was transmitted by very small bacteria which could not be seen under a microscope.

In 1892, Dmitri Iosifovich Ivanovsky, a Russian scientist, further discovered that by means of filtering bacteria, filtered sap from diseased tobacco leaves could still transfer bacteria to healthy leaves. He doubted the reliability of the filter. But, further research led him to conclude that there was a smaller microorganism permeating through the filters designed to trap ordinary bacteria.

In 1898, a Dutch scientist Martinus Beijerinck repeated the experiment with bacteria-free filtered extracts and confirmed that the infectious agents of the sap could reproduce themselves in infected tobacco leaves. He proposed that the etiological agent, smaller than bacteria, was the contagium vivum fluidum and named it "Virus," which could only survive in tobacco mosaic cells.

This is considered to be the beginning of virology.

In 1935, American scientist Wendell Meredith Stanley first isolated a needle-shaped crystal from tobacco leaves infected with tobacco mosaic disease and proved its ability to cause infection. He demonstrated that these viral particles composed of proteins were tobacco mosaic viruses.

British scientists Frederick Charles Bawden and Norman Wingate Pirie then discovered that the tobacco mosaic virus contained ribonucleic acid (RNA) composed of phosphorus

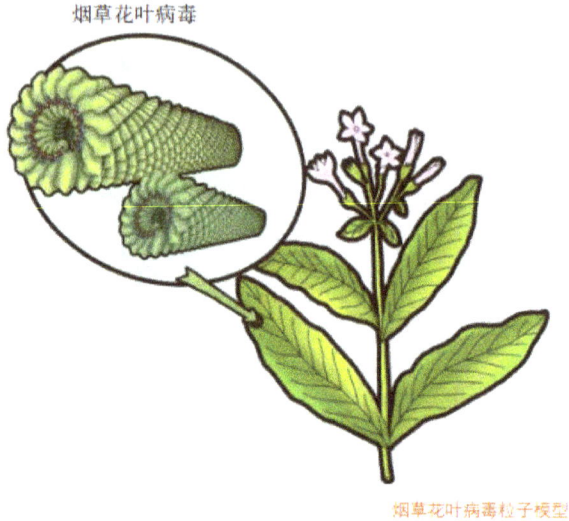

烟草花叶病毒

烟草花叶病毒粒子模型

Tobacco Mosaic Viruses and Tobacco Mosaic Virus Particle Model

and sugars. The RNA could be isolated from viral particles, demonstrating that the components of the virus were protein and nucleic acid.

In 1939, German scientist Gustav Adolf Kansche directly observed the tobacco mosaic virus under an electron microscope, a rod-shaped particle of 1.5 nm diameter and 300nm length. His studies further showed that the tobacco mosaic virus was a viral particle with a nucleic acid surrounded by a protein capsid.

But, human cognition is always circumscribed. Humans began to talk about "science" in recent years. It was not until 2005 that a modern technique — reverse genetics — was used by scientists to lift the veil from the 1918 flu virus.

It took 20 years for humans to realize the existence of viruses. But, we knew nothing about pathogens during the outbreak of the Great Flu. Thirteen years later, humans began to realize that is was the flu virus that caused the disease. Another five years later, the life components of the virus were identified. Then, seven years later, the visual evidence of the flu virus was obtained. The development of science and technology is the objective result of exploring nature, while the progress of science and technology can be subjectively used for social well-being. The flu virus was finally discovered, while the Great Flu just silently disappeared.

The first virus discovered by humans was the Tobacco Mosaic Virus (TMV). It was named "Mosaic" possibly due to the first impression left by its mysterious characteristics.

Can we do nothing but await our doom when facing the virus?

Chapter 3

The Story of the Cows

The milkmaids on the dairy farms in England set to work in the mist of the early morning. On their arms and hands were small scars due to cowpox, caused by their contact with cows, which did not affect their good mood because villages not far off were experiencing the case of the "smallpox." In the ancient East, inoculation was practiced in Chinese medicine.

1. Fight Poison with Poison

Viruses have known us long before we knew them.

Those who were born in China before the year of 1980 were likely to have thumbnail-sized scars on their arms. It was the mark of vaccination against smallpox, which China combated after witnessing an outbreak. In ancient times, people infected with smallpox would develop characteristic red rashes on their face, arms, and legs. The Greek named this disease as "the daughter of fire," while the Chinese called it "smallpox." The Kangxi Emperor of China's Qing Dynasty survived smallpox at a young age. The court painters of Qing Dynasty must have spent a lot of time modifying his portraits when he was infected with smallpox.

Smallpox, a fulminating infectious disease caused by the variola virus, is mainly spread through inhalation into the respiratory tract through sustained face-to-face contact between people. The main transmission mode is through aerosols consisting of airborne droplets from coughing or sneezing patients. In addition, the variola virus can spread through the fluid of the burst skin rash, or objects contaminated by them such as dust, clothing, food, and utensils.

The variola virus enters the body of susceptible people through the upper respiratory tract. It first attacks the mucous membrane of respiratory system, multiplies in the tonsil and other lymphatic tissues, and migrates into the bloodstream, resulting in temporary primary viremia. When the infected cell replicates and enters the bloodstream again, secondary viremia occurs.

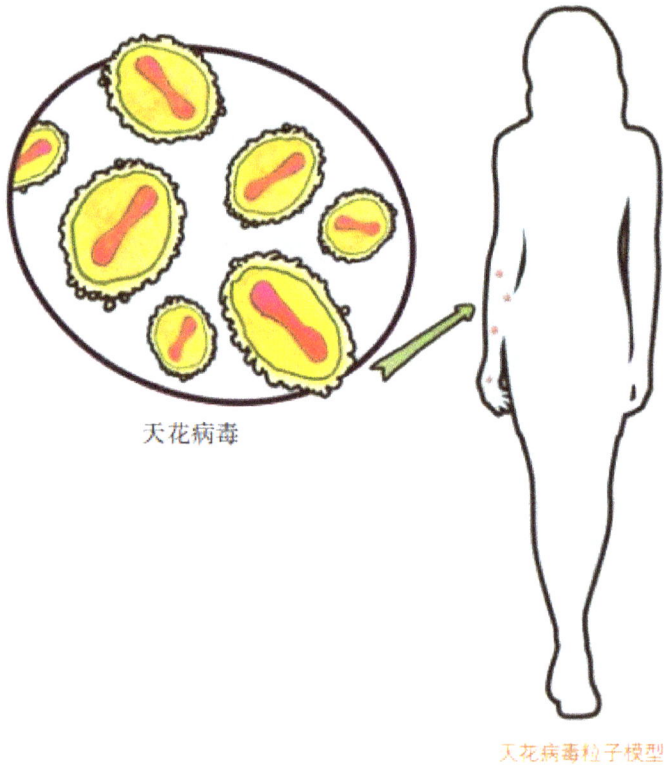

天花病毒

天花病毒粒子模型

The Variola Virus
The Variola Virus Particle Model

The virus can spread more widely through blood to the skin, mucous membranes, and internal organs of the body. After two to three days of its early symptoms, smallpox rash appears. Due to lack of heat tolerance, the viremia only lasts for a very short period, when the patient has a fever. Usually around a quarter of patients infected with smallpox will die. The flat and hemorrhagic smallpox are always fatal, since deaths often result from a profound toxemia or blood loss.

It is believed that smallpox, an ancient disease, appeared on Earth as early as 10,000 or 20,000 years ago. The first great plagues in human history such as the Plague of Athens, Antonine Plague, and American Plague, were almost closely related to the smallpox pandemic. In particular, complex chaos mixed with war, colonization, and disease occurred in the American continent in modern history, which pointed to one of the most dreadful diseases in human history: smallpox.

According to Chinese historical records, during the Jianwu period of Emperor Guangwu of Han Dynasty from 25–55 A.D., infected enemies captured brought smallpox to Nanyang. Thus, it was also called "the sore of the war prisoner." Introduced into China from abroad, smallpox became increasingly widespread in Tang and Song Dynasties, and even rampant in Yuan and Ming Dynasties. In the fight against smallpox, the ancient found those surviving smallpox could have a longer life expectancy, or even live to be 100 years old. Therefore, smallpox was also named "centenarian sore," which meant those infected could develop lifelong immunity to smallpox.

With the idea of "fighting poison with poison," some medical scientists developed variolation based on the above findings. Traditional Chinese medicine took the first step in the prevention and control of deadly smallpox. Sun Simiao, a famous physician in Tang Dynasty, introduced the mechanism of attacking the variola virus in his *Prescriptions Worth a Thousand Gold (Qianjin Yaofang)*, which was the earliest *Chinese Encyclopedia for Clinical Practice*. It could be deduced from the book that the variolation might be developed, but was only popular in civil society at that time.

Zhu Chunjia, a medical scientist in Qing Dynasty, wrote the story of Wang Dan, a famous minister of Song Dynasty, in *Conclusions of Smallpox (Douzhen Dinglun)*. Several sons and daughters of Wang Dan died due to smallpox. He had another son, Wang Su, in his old age. He searched everywhere for a skilled physician and prescriptions to protect his son from smallpox. Someone from Sichuan Province recommended a variolator in Mount Emei to him. Wang invited this variolator to Kaifeng upon hearing of him, who inoculated Wang Su the next day. On the seventh day, Wang Su developed a fever, and smallpox scab was formed 12 days later. Wang Su was free from smallpox as his father expected and lived until he was 67 years.

The methods of variolation developed by Chinese medical scientists are classified as follows:

Variolation through clothing: clothe a healthy person with the skirt of the child suffering from smallpox to infect him;

Wet variolation: place in a healthy child's nostril the vesicular fluid taken from a diseased child;

Dry variolation: pulverize scabs taken from smallpox sores and blow them into the nostrils of a healthy child;

Water variolation: pulverize and soak smallpox scabs in water, and then insert into the nose of an unaffected child.

However, our ancestors did not move beyond practical methods of "variolation" to corresponding theoretical hypotheses. Thus, they failed to establish the field of modern immunology.

The modern scientific method requires obtaining results in practice first, proposing a hypothesis by observing these results, verifying it in practice again, and continuous verification and practice until a complete scientific theory is formed.

The primitive wet variolation method was in fact developed to infect healthy persons with the variola virus to help them acquire immunity to smallpox. It is extremely hazardous since persons may be infected or killed by the variola virus, which was a "live vaccine" or smallpox agent directly taken from the infected.

This definitely proves the adage "nothing ventured, nothing gained." While there is nothing perfect in this world, as the saying goes "the stones of hills may be used to polish gems."

Edward Jenner discovered that a milkmaid infected with cowpox did not contract smallpox. People could become immune to smallpox by being vaccinated with cowpox. With deep thinking and exploration in his medical practice, he eventually succeeded in discovering a safer method to prevent smallpox.

2. Cowpox versus Smallpox

Smallpox spread in Europe in the 18th century, killing more than 150 million people in its wake. People at that time were so frightened of smallpox that they would turn pale at the mere mention of "pox." Thomas Babington Macaulay, a British historian, even termed smallpox "the accomplice of death."

In the autumn of 1798, Edward Jenner, an English doctor, introduced the idea of cowpox inoculation against smallpox in his paper "An Inquiry into the Cause and Effect of Variolae Vaccinae," in which 23 cases were described to prove the magic power of variolae vaccinae that those infected by it would never be attacked by smallpox even if the smallpox vesicular fluid was injected into their skin. In addition, the paper was also involved in the systematic demonstration of effects of cowpox inoculation against smallpox, morphological characteristics of variolae vaccinae, and such methods as vaccinia pulp and inoculation as well as vaccine reactions.

This was the first time in human history that cowpox inoculation was proven to prevent smallpox. At a time when everyone, including anxiety-stewed doctors and pain-stricken patients, could do nothing about the infectious smallpox spreading around the country, the following incident occurred Mr. Perkins, a neighbor of a milkmaid, was dying of smallpox. His wife, who had never been infected with smallpox, asked the milkmaid to take care of her husband. "Don't worry, Sir, I've taken care of several smallpox patients!" she said confidently.

It was a happy ending. He survived a bout with death although he bore scars on his face from the smallpox, while the milkmaid remained healthy after taking care of him.

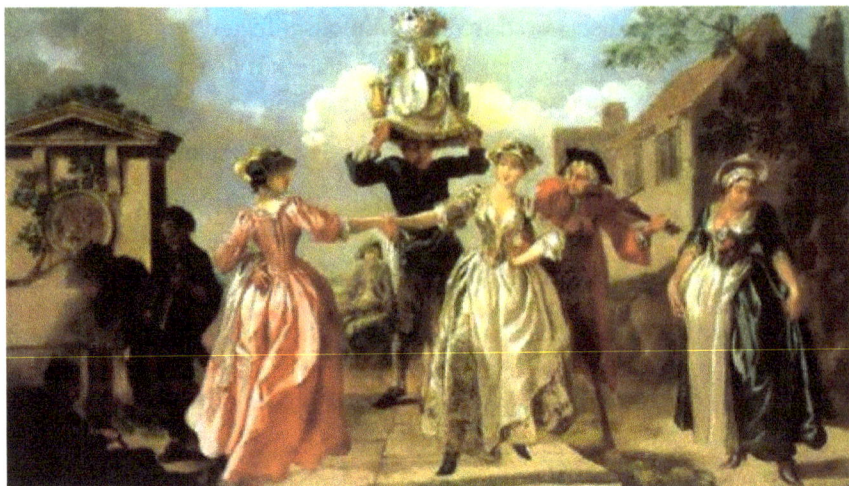

《挤奶女工的劳动节》油画

Oil Painting: *The Milkmaid's Garland*

It seemed that this incident inspired Dr. Jenner to figure out how to fight smallpox. He chatted with the milkmaid in detail and learned more about the prevailing cowpox and smallpox infection situation in the area from the other milkmaids. He gradually discovered clues to preventing smallpox and put forward a bold assumption that our body would acquire the immunity to smallpox if it was infected by cowpox, which meant smallpox could be prevented by the vaccine made from the vaccinia virus.

What a wonderful discovery it was! However, theory should be based on facts. Jenner, benefited from his previous rigorous medical training and began his experiments on animals. He found that, similar to infected humans, animals infected with cowpox remained alive. After his animal experiments, Jenner inoculated five cowpox-infected persons with smallpox vesicular fluid, none of whom contracted smallpox.

He then conducted a controlled trial with a more convincing finding: he vaccinated the experimental group consisting of 20 subjects who had been naturally infected with cowpox, and the control group with 20 subjects who had been infected by neither smallpox nor cowpox. It was found that the experimental group had no abnormal reactions, while the control group had severe symptoms such as fever and acne, and some of the subjects were even infected by smallpox.

Nevertheless, the finding remained widely doubted by the medical community at that time, since on one hand, this medical theory could not be verified by the technology then, and on the other hand, it was criticized and satirized by the religious community, and there were rumors that "people inoculated cowpox will develop cow-like appendages, such as horns on the head and cow-like voice."

The pursuit of truth is riddled with obstacles and failures. However, even a small step forward may light a spark for future of the human race.

With great trust and strong support of his family, Jenner inoculated his son. To continuously respond to doubts, he even conducted an open experiment:

Jenner gently scratched the arm of a boy who had never been infected with cowpox or smallpox and introduced into his skin a droplet of cowpox pus taken from the hand of a milkmaid infected with cowpox. A few days later, the boy developed a series of symptoms characteristic of cowpox inoculation. The boy recovered from cowpox two weeks later. To confirm the effect of cowpox inoculation, Jenner scratched the boy's arm with lethal infective pus that he had taken from a smallpox patient six weeks later, and found the boy did not come down with smallpox.

It took Jenner two years to wait for and observe the person naturally infected with cowpox for the sake of human safety. He did not report his findings to the public or officially declare smallpox could be conquered by humans until he verified this fact once more.

Subsequently, to prove cowpox inoculation could indeed be used for preventing smallpox, Jenner followed up his original publication with "Further Observation on the Variolae Vaccinae" in 1799 and "A Continuation of Facts and Observations Relative to the Variolae Vaccinae" in 1800. Those publications were soon translated into German, French, Dutch, Italian, and Latin and published worldwide. According to records, deaths from smallpox dropped by 92% in London, and smallpox infection and mortality rates were greatly reduced all over the world as a result of the wide application of Jenner's cowpox inoculation methods.

- In 1802, Jenner was granted £10,000 and a further £20,000 in 1807 for his achievement and the Royal Jennerian Society was established in London.
- From 1804 to 1814, two million people were vaccinated in Russia.
- In 1807, Bavaria made vaccination compulsory and celebrated Jenner's birthday as a holiday.
- From 1808 to 1811, 1.7 million people were vaccinated in France.
- From 1865 to 1885, 98.5% of the population was vaccinated in Italy.

The discovery by Jenner that "variolae vaccinae can be used to prevent smallpox," was popular across Europe and the Americas within a decade because it was simple and convenient while remaining safe and efficient.

The British government decreed that residents of all jurisdictions must be vaccinated and parents would be fined or jailed if they refuse to vaccinate their children. American President Thomas Jefferson resolutely sent vaccines to those in Virginia, his hometown, and all other parts of the America. Napoleon himself issued an order that all French troops who did not contract smallpox should be vaccinated.

From then on, variolae vaccinae was popular across the world, including China, where people got to know that variolae vaccinae could prevent smallpox after reading such works as *Yingjiliguo Xinchu Zhongdou Qishu* (*The Extraordinary History of a New Method of Inoculation Discovered in the Kingdom of England*, 1805) and *Yindou Lue* (*Introduction to the Extraction of the Cowpox Vaccine*, 1817). This new method of inoculation was extremely popular among the Chinese, and they never hesitate to accept this new method once they knew benefits it would bring to them.

The World Health Assembly began a global eradication campaign in 1959. In 1967, WHO officially launched an intensified plan to eradicate smallpox. Seventy million people were vaccinated in 19 countries of the West and Central Africa. Smallpox cases were only reported by only 31 countries in the world in 1968. By 1975, smallpox was eradicated from Asia. In 1980, WHO issued its official declaration that "the world and all its people have won freedom from smallpox."

Smallpox became the first plague conquered and its infectious agent, variola virus, was the first virus to be wiped out by humans.

"There were always scabs on our arms. They were the symbolic of variolae vaccinae, which helped us free from smallpox. Countless children have survived thanks to this vaccination." *Napoleon and Suina* (by Lu Xun, a famous Chinese liltterateur, 1935, the transliterated name of "Jenner" was "Suina").

The discovery that "Variolae vaccinae protects people from smallpox" is regarded as a milestone in immunology. Vaccinia, a weak strain of poxvirus that is less harmful than smallpox, can help our bodies develop immunity to smallpox. Based on this discovery, scientists established the theoretical framework of "cellular immunity" and "humoral immunity," paving the way ahead for further design and discovery of novel vaccines and drugs.

3. Apocalypse

Jenner succeeded in conquering smallpox. More importantly, he discovered the approach to enabling humans to prevent diseases with their unique immune system. He inspired scientists to make unremitting efforts in the prevention and treatment of infectious diseases by laying the foundation for development of smallpox prevention and pointing the way to combating other diseases. Jenner, who was later honored as "the great scientific discoverer and life saver" and "the father of immunology," successfully ushered in a new field — immunology.

Originating from medical science and early studies on diseases, immunology is a discipline that studies the structure and function of the immune system, which helps humans realize their unique immunity. It was not until the 18th century that the mysteries of the immune system were eventually revealed step by step by the concerted efforts of several generations of scientists.

With the development of microbiology, Pasteur produced vaccines from weakened anthrax bacteria and attenuated viruses in rabies by the end of the 19th century. Their effectiveness in conferring immunity has been proved when pioneers developed these vaccines. However, several uncertainties and unknowns remain about how vaccines work and what the immune system does to protect the body from pathogen invasion.

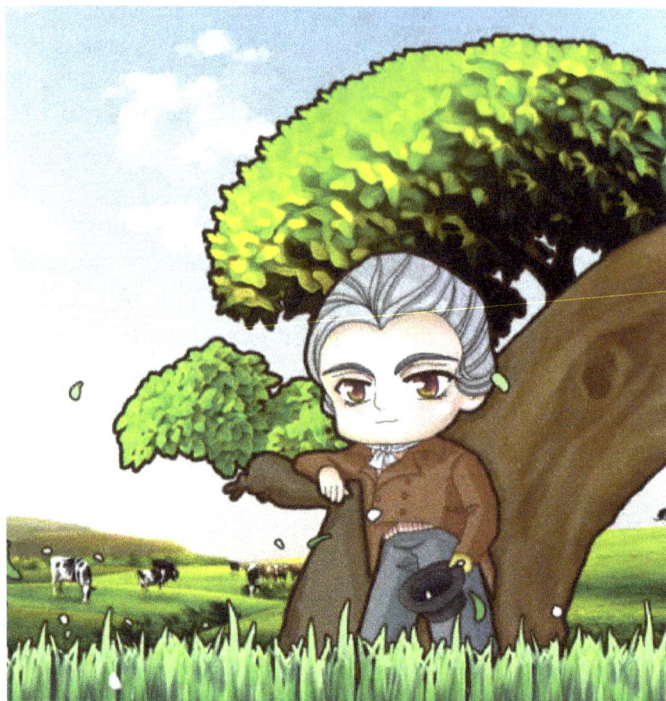

爱德华·琴纳医生

Doctor Edward Jenner

"Cellular Immunity" and "Humoral Immunity"

Ilya Ilyich Mechnikov, a Russian zoologist, and Paul Ehrlich, a German immunologist, made great achievements in determining the immune mechanism of antibodies. They established the concepts of "cellular immunity" and "humoral immunity," respectively, which provided a theoretical framework for addressing complex immune system problems. Immunology has developed into an independent discipline since then.

In 1883, when he was dissecting a leech, Mechnikov discovered that food could be "swallowed" directly by its intestinal cells. He then discovered that in embryos of coelenterates such as hydra, siphonophores, and hydromedusae, their digestive system was not a sac but a tube, and concluded that in the process of evolution, food could be directly taken into cells for animals without an obvious digestive tract to absorb nutrients.

In addition to studying the digestive tracts of animals, he also observed some swimming phagocytic cells under a microscope, which could "eat" tadpole-like tails of senescent or metamorphic cells. He called them "macrophages" in 1883.

He then proved foreign invaders could be cleared by the defense system comprising macrophages, lymphocytes, and other tissues by observing starfish and water fleas in his experiment. Macrophages "eat" not only senescent cells in humans but also invading pathogenic microbes such as bacteria to protect the body. Mechnikov then established a systematic theory of cellular immunity based on his further studies.

Paul Ehrlich, a German immunologist, participated in developing an antiserum for treating tetanus and diphtheria in 1889, during which he proposed that fundamental differences of disparate tissues and cells could cause different responses to foreign substances such as dyes or bacterial toxins.

Paul Ehrlich proposed the well-known "side-chain theory" in 1897. Antigens, which refer to bacteria, viruses, protein toxins, foreign animal serums, and others entering the human body, have binding sites and special "side chains," namely "binding clusters." Antibodies, which refer to substances produced due to stimulation by antigens to help defend the body against foreign invasion, also have "side chains" or "binding clusters." Due to their special chemical properties, "binding clusters" of certain antibodies must be matched to "binding clusters" of their correspondent antigens as "locks and keys."

The body can clear antigens or deprive their pathogenic functions through interactions between "binding clusters" of antibodies and antigens. Some antibodies stimulated by specific antigens bind directly to them, while the rest protect the body from specific invading antigens via the circulating blood and fluids throughout the body. Ehrlich first demonstrated the immune process according to the antibody theory and chemical response, and established the systematic theory of humoral immunity.

Three Lines of Defense

Mechnikov and Ehrlich helped people understand the immune system by explaining how vaccine works in a scientific manner. Human body relies on the immune system to recognize "self" and "not self" and maintain homeostasis. There are "three lines of defense" to defend human bodies against external invaders:

- The first line of defense, composed of skin and mucous membranes of the body, acts as exterior walls of the castle to block and shield pathogens outside from entering the body. Foreign substances and pathogens can be cleared in the interaction of human body and environment with the help of bactericidal substances such as stomach acid and enzymes produced by skins and mucous membranes and the protective cilia on the surface of respiratory mucosa.
- The second line of defense refers to natural immune systems such as phagocytes and killer cells in the body, which act as standing armies defending the castle. Once the first line of defense, such as skin or mucous membranes, is broken by pathogens, phagocytes will rush out of capillaries and gather in pathogen-infected areas to engulf them, and natural killer cells will destroy pathogen activity or lyse infected cells by producing and releasing perforins and cytokines. Under general conditions, the second line of defense can resist invasion of common pathogens and eliminate majority of their hostile provocations.
- The third line of defense is the specific immune system consisted of lymphocytes such as T lymphocytes and B lymphocytes, which act as special forces of the praetorian guard. When the first and second lines of defense have been broken, the body's immune system will become so alert that immune cells will be sent to carefully study invaders and carry out targeted training and arming. Killer T cells with "special martial arts skills" will be activated, and B cells will be required to manufacture special antibody "weapons." They are the so-called specific cellular immunity and humoral immunity, "working along both lines" to fight against enemies in the body.

If the immune system wins, the body keeps healthy, whereas if bacteria and viruses win, they will cause disease in the body.

Natural immunity is non-specific, which means it can resist invasions of a variety of pathogenic microorganisms, but with relatively weak resistance to infectious agents. Acquired immunity is specific, which can produce a relatively strong protection against a specific pathogen after being stimulated by specific microbial antigens.

Vaccines are also antigenic substances similar to those in bacteria or viruses. Specific antibodies will be produced after inoculation with resistance to specific bacteria or viruses. Infectious diseases will not be caused due to dead or attenuated virulence in the vaccine. Inoculation is an artificial way to stimulate the special active immunity in the body's immune system.

Jenner discovered the vaccinia virus in nature, which was harmless to humans and could help the body to produce immunity to smallpox virus, and thus was known as the weakened vaccine; whereas the rabies vaccine, developed by Pasteur through multiple artificial passages and drying methods to attenuate its pathogenicity so as to help the body produce immunity to the rabies virus, was known as the attenuated vaccine.

Jenner and Pasteur made great contributions to human health with their careful observations and patient work in experiments, though scientific theories of vaccine prevention remained unknown to them at that time.

Science ushered in a new starting point with the development of immunology from then on and the establishment of virology 100 years later.

Do we have to resort to nothing but observations and experiments when solving problems?

Chapter 4

The World of Molecules

Many life science and medical theories have been discovered and recognized through scientific and technological breakthroughs. Particularly, the discovery of the DNA double helix has allowed humans to explore the inner mysteries of cells such as genetic materials and proteins, leading to the molecular research evolution in genetic engineering.

1. Life Pool

Life science is like a great ocean filled with countless treasures and mysteries. We can hardly describe how magnificent the ocean of life science is. Let us enjoy the "ripples" of the micro-molecular world left by the surging "rivers."

However, the world is so big while molecules are so small. How can we explore them?

You are right! Just follow your instinct and study yourself. We, humans, should know everything about ourselves.

Humans are multicellular organisms, and viruses are hosts in cells. Human cells and viruses are made of proteins and nucleic acids, the former acting as functional carriers of life and the latter the genetic materials of life.

Thus, let us explore life's mysteries by studying the five key levels of our body with the "basic reduction method."

The First Level: Human Body

The human body is composed of the respiratory system, digestive system, motor system, immune system, blood system, and other systems, jointly performing normal physiological functions of the body. For example, the respiratory system acts as the site for gas exchange by consuming oxygen and producing carbon dioxide; the digestive system helps the body to obtain nutrition from food and use it for energy; and the motor system mainly maintains motor functions by supporting and protecting the body.

The system is the combination of multiple organs with one or more physiological functions in a certain order; the organ is made of different tissues to perform specific functions for the body; the tissue is a group of

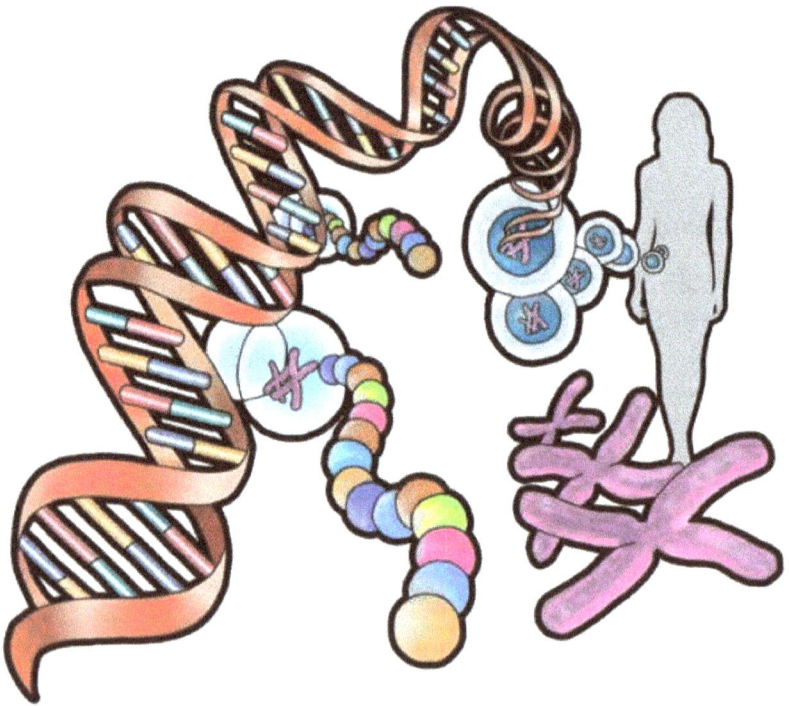

生命五重要素之"还原基本法"：人、细胞、病毒、蛋白质、核酸

Five Levels of Life with the "Basic Reduction Method": Human Body, Cell, Virus, Protein, and Nucleic Acid.

cells sharing the same morphological features and functions; and the cell is the basic functional unit of life.

The human blood circulatory system mainly consists of bone marrow, thymus, lymph nodes, spleen, other tissues and organs, as well as blood cells throughout the body, mainly red blood cells, white blood cells, and platelets. As the structural and functional unit of the human body, the total number of cells is 40–60 trillion.

The red blood cell is the major carrier of oxygen and carbon dioxide. It is red because of the hemic iron ions in the hemoglobin. The white blood cell is colorless, and its major function is fighting bacteria and viruses and maintaining human immunity. White blood cells can be divided according to their morphological differences based on the presence or absence of granules. Platelets, which are cell fragments derived from mature megakaryocytes of the bone marrow, mainly perform such functions as hemostasis and tissue repair.

The white blood cell can be further divided into neutrophils, basophils, eosinophils, monocytes, and lymphocytes.

Neutrophils and monocytes play an important role in defending the human body by engulfing bacteria and foreign invading pathogens. Neutrophils can also produce phagocytin and lysozyme to eliminate pathogens, and activated monocytes can "transform" into macrophages with a stronger phagocytic function.

Basophils contain basophil granules, which can rapidly release anti-coagulant heparin and histamine in allergic reactions. Eosinophils can attenuate allergic reactions by releasing histaminase to inactivate histamine. Moreover, they can bind to surfaces of certain parasites via their antibodies and release substances from their granules that kill them.

Lymphocytes can be further divided into NK cells, T lymphocytes, and B lymphocytes. While NK cells can kill target cells non-specifically, T cells can specifically and directly kill target cells or assist B cells in producing antibodies, and stimulated by antigens, B cells can differentiate into plasma cells, which synthesize and secrete specific antibodies.

What are antibodies? This question will be answered in the fourth level: "basic reduction method."

The Second Level: Cell

In 1665, Robert Hooke, an English physicist, coined the term "cell" for describing the microscopical pores he observed in plant cells — more precisely, cell walls in a clean cork tissue, similar to a honey-comb.

As the smallest structural and functional unit of an organism, the cell is the basic physical unit for growth and development of life, just as sand acts as the basic unit of a sea shore and brick the basic unit of a building. Cells are tiny, measuring 10–30 micrometers in diameter, and can be observed under an optical microscope.

Single-celled organisms can carry out all life functions on their own; while in multicellular organisms, each cell has a relatively independent life though the organisms' functions are coordinated and controlled as a whole. Generally, most microorganisms like bacteria and protozoans like paramecium and amoeba are single-celled organisms, while plants such as metasequoia and phoenix trees and animals like lions and humans are multicellular organisms.

The multicellular organism keeps replacing aging and dying cells with nascent ones so as to maintain its metabolism or repair tissue damage even if it has completed its development. Around 100 million cells die every minute throughout the human body. There are 200 to 300 types of cells with different sizes and shapes in the human body.

In the micro world, the cell, as a structural and functional unit, is a collection of smaller biomolecules. For example, certain amounts of organic macromolecules, such as nucleic acids, proteins, polysaccharides, and lipids, form subcelluar structures in a precise manner. These functional and morphological subcellular structures are organelles, including mitochondria and ribosomes, which eventually make up cells.

A large number of complex biochemical and metabolic activities take place in organelles during the cell cycle. The nucleus, a closed membranous organelle in a eukaryotic cell, contains most of the genetic material (DNA and RNA) of a cell. The mitochondria are uniformly distributed in the cytosol of plant and animal cells and serve as the important source of energy for cells. The chloroplast, an organelle only found in plant cells, serves as the site of plant cell photosynthesis, through which the light energy is converted into chemical energy of plants. Endoplasmic reticulum is responsible for the transport of materials from the nucleus to cytoplasm, cell membrane, and outside the cell. Ribosome is the site of a cell in which protein synthesis takes place. Golgi apparatus is an organelle involved in protein process and transport.

In short, all organelles work to achieve continuous cell transmission from one generation to the next, which is a process of constant renewal.

The cell "rebooting" process occurs together with its division. The life of a cell begins with its formation by cell division of a mother cell and ends either with the formation of daughter cells or with its death. The cell cycle generally refers to the period between the beginning of one cell division to the beginning of next, during which the replicated genetic material of a mother cell is distributed equally and identically into two daughter cells.

From the perspective of its functions, there are two cell division types: one is for cell replication, including binary fission, mitosis, and amitosis, etc., during which the genetic material remains the same after the cell division and new cell cycle begins; the other is cytogenetic division, such as meiosis in germ cells, during which only half the number of chromosomes in new cells wait to be matched those from another cell and continue the next cell cycle.

Cell division is not necessarily a strict "one to one" model. Cells in different conditions may have divisions with "multiple identities," exhibiting a state of "self-release." For example, yeast can undergo such divisions as dichotomy, mitosis, amitosis, budding, and spore reproduction. It is the virus in an organism that is more difficult to be observed than the cell.

The above-mentioned obscure cellular "components" will be used for explaining the following viral "widgets."

The Third Level: Virus

A virus is an infectious agent that must use cell processes to replicate. A common virus consists of nucleic acid and a protein capsid. Nucleic acid, which is the center of a virus, stores genetic information. The protein capsid, surrounding the nucleic acid, mediates the binding of a virus to a host cell. A virus is a "weirdo" only inside the living cells of an organism.

One can say the life course is the cell history, while it is impossible to regard the cell history as the virus history.

Did life really get started with electrical sparks in the "Miller experiment"? Or is it an alien life form surviving in the wreckage after an extraterrestrial body hit the earth?

This is a question that is yet to be answered.

At present, there are three major hypotheses about the origin of virus:

- The first hypothesis is called the regressive hypothesis or degeneracy theory. It suggests that viruses were once small cells that parasitized larger cells. As time went by, genes not required by their parasitism were lost. The essence of this theory is "the cells losing part of their functions."
- The second hypothesis is called cellular origin hypothesis or vagrancy hypothesis, which states that viruses evolved from bits of RNA or DNA that escaped from the genes of larger organisms. The essence of this theory is "they are part of cells' functions."
- The third hypothesis is called coevolution hypothesis or virus-first hypothesis, which states that viruses evolved from complex molecules of protein and nucleic acid at the same time as the first cells appeared on earth billions of years ago. They have been dependent on cellular life ever since. The essence of this theory is "viruses came before cells or cells and viruses evolved alongside each other."

A controversial statement about the origin of life on earth is that "life began with viruses." The supporting argument is that viruses are the simplest forms of precellular life; while the opposing argument is that viruses do not functionally meet conditions of the simplest precellular life.

This is certainly another problem.

Viruses are often described as "organisms on the edge of life," since viruses with (nucleic acid) genes can evolve by natural selection and replicate themselves through self-assembly as other organisms. However, without cellular structures, viruses, even with nucleic acid, cannot survive independently but have to live in a living cell to complete its life cycle.

Viruses are usually smaller than cells, but larger than most biological macromolecules. The size of a typical virus is 100 nanometers, and a cell is 10 micrometers or 10,000 nanometers, which also explains why a virus can parasitize in a cell from a spatial perspective. There are exceptions on the size. For example, ancient **Pandoraviruses**, discovered by French scientists in Siberian permafrost in 2013, are 1,000 nanometers in diameter, whose host is the **Amoeba** that is 50,000 nanometers (50 micrometers) in diameter.

The life cycle of a virus includes six stages: attachment, penetration, uncoating, biosynthesis, assembly, and release, which is closely related to the above-mentioned cell life cycle. Without replication functions, viruses have to replicate themselves during the cell replication. Therefore, the key is how to control the cell "components" to produce virus "widgets" in a cell life cycle.

Attachment: viruses infecting humans can be divided into two types based on their surface structures: (1) enveloped viruses with the lipid bilayer derived from host cell membranes and (2) non-enveloped viruses. The glycoproteins spikes, protruding on the external membrane of a typical enveloped virus, can bind to specific receptor proteins in the outer membrane of a host cell, leading to the attachment of the virus to the host cell. The non-enveloped virus also has protein molecules on its surface to bind to the host cell.

Penetration: when the virus attaches to the host cell, it will open the outer membrane to enter the cell. Some types of enveloped virus are engulfed as a whole by endocytosis, whereas others fuse directly into the cell's membrane. Most viruses enter the cytoplasm of host cells, while some enter their nuclei.

Uncoating: after entering the host cell and removing their capsid, some viruses release the genetic material and integrate them to the genome of the host cell's nucleus. Then, they rewrite genetic information instructions and encode their genetic information to the cellular genetic library, while other viruses release genetic material from the membrane to the cytoplasm and encode their own genetic information.

Biosynthesis: organelles in a cell will produce and replicate the genetic material and proteins for viruses according to the genetic information they modified. Such organelles as ribosomes and golgiosomes thus become manufacturing factories providing raw material for assembling new viruses.

Assembly: after the biosynthesis of genetic material and proteins, viruses will make use of their protease to process and modify "widgets" for their assembly to endow them with biological activity of viruses.

Release: with the nucleic acid and protease surrounded by the capsid obtained from cell endoplasmic reticulum and membrane (enveloped viruses), new infectious virions come into being and leave the cell to complete their life cycle.

These six stages not only affect cell reproduction and consume cellular resources as well as energies, but also damage the normal physiological functions of cells. Meanwhile, more viruses will be produced after replication, which will further infect other host cells and then affect tissues, organs, and overall functions of the organism.

After understanding basic forms of life such as human body, cells, and viruses, let us explore basic matters of life.

Do you feel a little bit excited to read the following sections?

The Fourth Level: Protein

In 1838, Gerardus Johannes Mulder, a Dutch chemist, extracted the common substance from animal tissues and plant sap. He found that almost all of them have the same chemical composition and that living organisms could not survive without them. The substance is protein, derived from a Greek word *protos* meaning "primary or first."

You must disagree that protein is the most abundant substance in human body since water is the source of all life. But protein accounts for 45% of human body's total solids and 75% of muscle tissues if water is excluded. Protein is the basic component of skin, muscle, heart, hair, blood, and bones. It is made up of amino acids.

As the embodiment of macromolecules and life activities, protein is not only the basic substance of cells and organisms, but also an important regulator of their metabolism. Proteins are part of every cell, tissue, and organ in human bodies. They are fundamental elements providing nutrients for the growth and development of body. Proteins in such plant seeds as beans, peanuts, and wheat or in meat and cheese are sources of essential nutrients for an organism's growth.

Protein is the executor of biological structure and physiological function. For example, human hair, nails, and animal feathers are mainly composed of keratin, which protects and supports bodies; skin is mainly made up of collagen and keratin, among which, the former can maintain the shape and structure of skin and keep it firm and supple; hemoglobin, the protein inside red blood cells, is responsible for transporting oxygen and carbon dioxide; and the salivary enzyme amylase catalyzes the hydrolysis of food starch into maltose.

Proteins are essential for maintaining health and preventing diseases. They are major components in active substances in human body such as enzymes, hormones, and antibodies; insulin, the only hormone lowering blood sugar in the body, can promote glycogen, fat, and protein synthesis and be used to treat diabetes; antibodies can enable humans to resist the invasion of diseases and external pathogens by identifying and binding to foreign proteins, viruses, and bacteria to eliminate harmful particles entering the body.

An antibody is an immunoglobulin Y (IgY) produced by mature B lymphocytes for neutralizing pathogens. It is a monomer with a symmetrical structure consisting of four polypeptide chains: two identical longer heavy chains with more molecules and two identical shorter light chains with less molecules connected by disulfide bonds and non-covalent bonds.

An antigen is any substance stimulating an immune response. It can be either a protein or a non-protein, and a living substance or a non-living one. Usually most antigens such as proteins, bacteria, and viruses can cause immune responses in human body to produce specific antibodies.

Certain toxic proteins can serve as important weapons for animals to attack enemies and protect themselves. Most animal toxins are proteins. They can cause damage to body's functions after entering the body, including respiratory failure caused by the blocked transmission of nerve excitation, local or systemic bleeding caused by broken capillaries, severe muscle necrosis, and poisoning or death of animals and humans.

Venom proteins secreted from the venom gland of a venomous snake can kill its prey; and worker bees can protect themselves in the face of a threat by secreting an aromatic protein-rich liquid. Varied in shapes and functions, proteins are very important for the body. What are secrets of nucleic acids in nuclei of cells or viral protein particles of viruses?

The Fifth Level: Nucleic Acid

Gregor Mendel, an Austrian priest, discovered the fundamental laws of inheritance through his crossbreeding experiment on pea plants in 1865, which laid the foundation for modern genetics. He concluded that genetic factors controlling the same trait (like pea plant height) exist in pairs in somatic cells of the organism, and they separate and enter different gametes, passing down to the offspring. As an old saying goes, "As a man sows, so shall he reap."

Friedrich Miescher, a Swiss scientist, collected a large number of surgical bandages from nearby hospitals. He discovered a strong organic acid with larger amounts of phosphorus than those in proteins by dividing cells from the serum and other substances in the pus on those surgical bandages. He then named this strong organic acid as nucleic acid.

Cell is the fundamental unit of life activity, with proteins and nucleic acid serving as its basic components. Nucleic acids and proteins, which are both called biological macromolecules, are carriers of biological genetic information. They play crucial roles in genetic variation and protein synthesis. The basic unit of a nucleic acid is a nucleotide. Nucleic acid can be divided into two categories: deoxyribonucleic acid (DNA) and ribonucleic acid (RNA).

James Dewey Watson, an American geneticist, and Francis Crick, a British crystallographer, determined the double-helix structure of DNA in 1953. DNA, with the double helix structure, is a biological molecule in nature that can replicate itself. The fine and accurate self-replication of DNA ensures ancestors' biological traits to be passed on to their next generation.

Similar to "two dragons playing with pearls," the two main strands of DNA, parallel but opposite to each other, spiral around the same axis in the right-hand helix to form the double helix configuration. With its "simple beauty," its structure has become the hallmark of modern biology. Anyone who sees the DNA model will feel excited and make the following remark "such a beautiful structure exists ."

The discovery of the DNA double helix structure ushered in a new era of molecular biology, when biomacromolecules can be studied at a new research stage and genetics can be explored at the molecular level. This is an important step in understanding "the mystery of life" as well as a landmark in life science in the 20th century.

In 1957, a British scientist Francis Crick put forward the Central Dogma, which holds that genetic information flows in the direction DNA $\rightarrow$ RNA $\rightarrow$ protein. It is stated that genetic information is transcribed from DNA to RNA and then translated from mRNA to protein. Subsequent studies found that proteins can also assist in the transcription and translation and contribute to DNA genetic functions.

As the fundamental dogma of transfer of genetic information between different biomacromolecules, the Central Dogma enables humans to decipher the "code of life." It is like a programmer who urgently stores the information of all living things in the sophisticated world after mastering the source code of programming. He starts up the program to run these information codes, only to find the information chain is a complete system with different feedback loops. Each type of living system is a miracle of creation, with each loop in it deciphering codes and each system working to build a sound model. Some examples are as follows:

- The Human Genome Project (HGP): 23 pairs of chromosomes and 20,000 to 30,000 genes.
- The Human Microbiome Project (HMP): there are about 10 times as many microbial cells in the human body as there are human cells, containing about 100 times as many genes as the human genome.
- The Global Virome Project (GVP): to discover a million unknown viruses.

While creating a miracle is the dream of all human beings, let us set a small goal first.

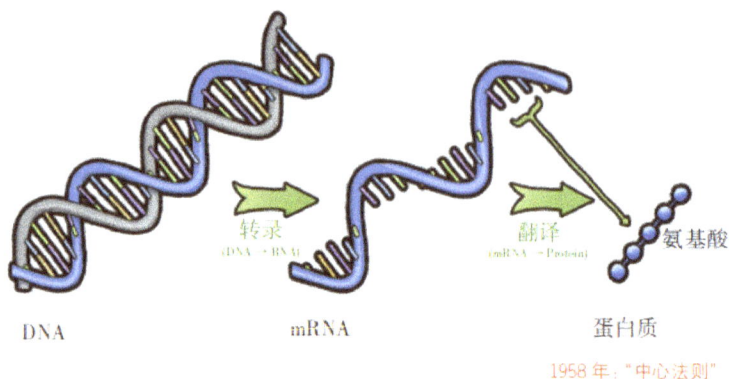

DNA Transcription → mRNA Translation → Protein → Amino Acid

1958: The Central Dogma

With the development of modern biological techniques such as polymerase chain reaction (PCR), hybridoma cell lines, stem cells, electron microscope, and the establishment of upgraded platforms such as the high-level biosafety laboratory, favorable conditions have been created to explore the microscopic world and cutting-edge tools have been provided to develop and utilize biological resources.

2. Microbes in the Surging Sea

Question One: How to See a Virus?

Antony van Leeuwenhoek, a Dutch scientist, made his own optical microscope with such rare and precious materials as gems, diamonds, and glass in the 17th century to observe a microscopic world in dust, water droplets, blood, insects, and plants for the first time. He then made various lenses, some of which provided magnification of up to 300 times. He referred to microbes observed under the optical microscope as *Dierken*, namely, "the tiny and animated things."

We can hear a sound because of sound waves. Similarly, we can see an object because of light waves. Visible light, the only one that can be perceived by human eyes, has wavelengths in the range of 400–760 nanometers. Therefore, it can be deduced based on this data that bacteria rather than viruses can be captured under an optical microscope since the most sophisticated one has a resolution of less than 200 nanometers.

The lens principle of the optical microscope follows the wave-particle duality principle of light. In 1905, Einstein proposed that light has dual properties of wave and a particle. In 1924, De Broglie put forward the theory of "matter wave," which holds that all matters have wave and particle duality and electrons also have such wave-like phenomena as interference and diffraction, which was further confirmed by the electron diffraction experiment.

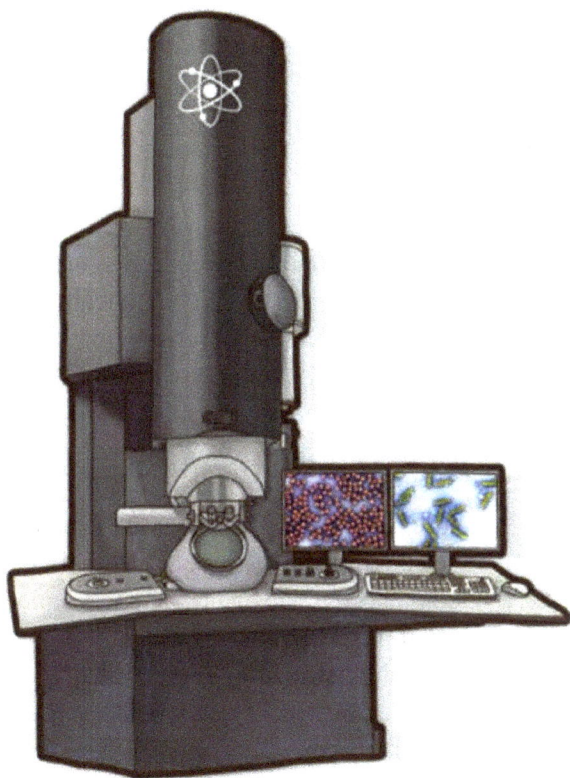

电子显微镜模型图

Electron Microscope

In short, electrons can do what the light can do. But can electrons do what the light cannot do?

An electron is a small negatively charged particle outside the nucleus. The "electric" ring enables people to use electromagnetic fields to speed up electrons, resulting in a much shorter wavelength. Similar to the light focusing in an optical microscope, a higher resolution can be achieved by focusing a high-speed electron beam.

Ernst Ruska and Max Knoll built the first electron lens in 1931; the resolution was improved up to 50 nanometers in 1934; the resolution of the high-resolution electron microscope was achieved up to 3 nanometers in 1939; the resolution of scanning tunneling microscope (STM) was 0.01 nanometers in 1978, with the distance between two minimum resolvable points being one-tenth of the atom diameter. The electron is once again studied from the perspective of atom.

1 m = 1000 mm
1 mm = 1000 um
1 um = 1000 nm
1 nm = 10 Å

The development of high-resolution microscopy enables us to clearly see the outside of virus as well as its inside components such as proteins and nucleic acids. The extremely fast electrons endow us with a "smart eye" to solve the "morph" problem on a micro scale of life.

Question Two: How to Obtain Genetic Information from Viruses?

The double helix structure of DNA and the Central Dogma lay a theoretical foundation for molecular biology. There are four different Bases in DNA: Adenine (A), Guanine (G), Cytosine (C), and Thymine (T) — "A," "G," "C," and "T" for short, respectively.

The periphery of the DNA structure, composed of phosphoric acid and pentose, is supported by the energy provided by the phospholipid bond. The reverse double helix structure inside DNA, with the pairing model of four Bases of A, G, C, T, namely, the base pair principle of A=T and G=C, is stabilized by the molecular force of the hydrogen bond.

It Is far from enough to see life forms if we want to carry out research on life science. The research on genetic information is a desirable breakthrough point in understanding the nature of life. Now here is the next question: a large amount of biological materials has to be cultured and consumed to obtain the nucleic acids from cells or viruses if the washing-bandage method continues to be used for extraction. Is it possible to directly replicate and amplify targeted DNA pieces and study life at the molecular level?

It is easy to change from "big" to "small," but difficult from "less" to "more." If A, T, G, and C bases are combined one by one and linked together according to their chemical properties, it must be costly and time-consuming as well as labor-consuming.

The semi-reserved mode of DNA replication is an important way for biological evolution and passage. Double-stranded DNA, which is affected by different types of enzymes, can be denatured and unwound into single strands. With the participation of DNA polymerase, the same two DNA molecules will be copied by complementary base-pairing.

Consequently, the DNA double helix structure separates into two complementary single-stranded DNAs. Affected by a certain nucleic acid polymerase, uncoiled single-stranded DNA acts as a template to synthesize new complementary single strand DNA according to the four base pairing principle, and the reaction will repeat at a logarithmic level, eventually establishing the automatic assembly system with an "assembly line."

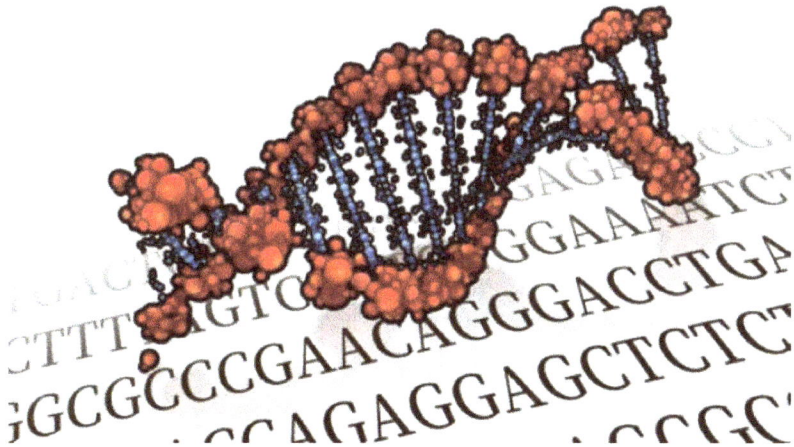

DNA "密码子"：腺嘌呤（A）、鸟嘌呤（G）、胞嘧啶（C）、胸腺嘧啶（T）

DNA "Codons": Adenine (A), Guanine (G), Cytosine (C), and Thymine (T)

The basic principle is polymerase chain reaction (PCR).

The PCR technique ushers in a channel to obtain and apply nucleic acid molecules . Humans can study viruses through their genetic information or structures and functions of their proteins. However, the central theme remains the same, that ultimately live viruses must be studied, which is a dangerous cause.

Question Three: How to Ensure Safety in Studying Viruses?

Robert Koch, a German bacteriologist, was the pioneer and founder of pathogenic bacteriology and put forward the classic "Koch's postulates." He is considered as the "plague buster" for his contributions in the first discovery of *Bacillus Anthracis* and *Vibrio Cholerae* and succeeded in performing the first isolation of typhoid bacillus and *Mycobacterium tuberculosis*, and his method of pure culture of bacteria with solid media. In 1886, he published a report on the laboratory-acquired cholerae infection, which was supposed to be the first report on biosafety in the world.

In the 1940s, people began to attach great importance to laboratory-acquired infection throughout the world. US built the first biosafety laboratory and issued the standard of *Classification of Etiologic Agents on the Basis of Hazard* in 1974, in which four hazard levels were first divided according to pathogenic microorganisms available to be studied and corresponding activities conducted in the laboratory. In the 1980s, WHO rated biosafety laboratories from level 1 to level 4. Pathogenic microorganisms refer to microbes that have the potential to invade human body and cause infections or infectious diseases. They are also called pathogens. Bacteria and viruses are the most dangerous pathogens. Infection can be defined as the process in which pathogens in host cells grow, reproduce, and release toxic substances that lead to pathogenic changes and even death of the body. The hazard degree of pathogenic microorganisms declines from level 1 to level 4 according to the classification criteria in China, while it increases according to those of WHO and foreign countries.

Pathogenic microorganisms categorized in Level 1 are microbes that cause the most severe diseases in humans and animals or those undiscovered or declared extinct in China.

Pathogenic microorganisms categorized in Level 2 refer to microbes causing severe diseases in humans and animals and ordinarily spread from humans to humans, animals to humans, and animals to animals.

Pathogenic microorganisms categorized in Level 3 are microbes causing diseases in humans and animals with limited harms to humans, animals, or environment on general conditions. With the moderate risk of transmission, it is hard to cause severe diseases after the laboratory-acquired infection and effective treatment and preventive measures are available.

Pathogenic microorganisms categorized in Level 4 are microbes unlikely to cause diseases in humans or animals on general conditions.

Biosafety Laboratories are those biological or animal laboratories which meet biosafety requirements. They can avoid or control harmful biological agents with protective barriers and management measures. Laboratory Biosafety Level (BSL; or Protection, P) can be divided from level 1 to level 4. BSL-1 is fundamental to laboratories of all biosafety levels and BSL-4 are those of highest biosafety levels, which are consistent with international categorizations of pathogenic microorganisms but opposite to those in China.

BSL-1 laboratories: microorganisms handled at this level are unlikely to cause diseases in human or animals, namely microbes of BSL-1 (or pathogenic microorganisms categorized in Level 4, such as measles virus, mumps virus, etc.).

BSL-2 laboratories: microorganisms handled at this level are those causing diseases in humans and animals but with limited harms to humans, animals, or environment on general conditions. With the moderate risk of transmission, it is hard to cause severe diseases after the laboratory-acquired infection and effective treatment and preventive measures are available, namely microbes of BSL-2 (or pathogenic microorganisms categorized in Level 3, such as *Staphylococcus aureus*, hepatitis B virus, etc.).

BSL-3 laboratories: microorganisms handled at this level are those causing severe diseases in humans and animals and ordinarily spread from

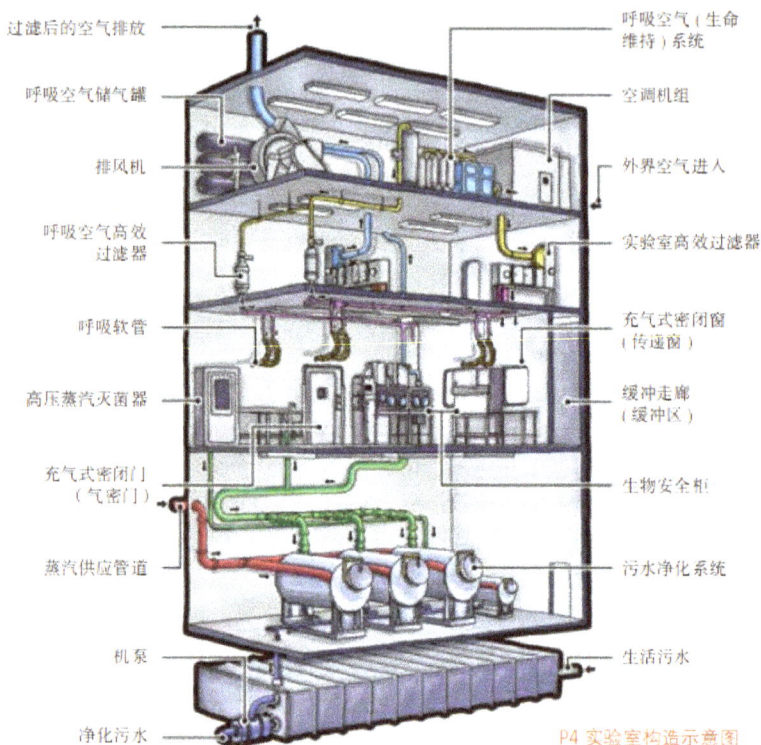

过滤后的空气排放 — 呼吸空气（生命维持）系统

呼吸空气储气罐 — 空调机组

排风机 — 外界空气进入

呼吸空气高效过滤器 — 实验室高效过滤器

呼吸软管 — 充气式密闭窗（传递窗）

高压蒸汽灭菌器 — 缓冲走廊（缓冲区）

充气式密闭门（气密门） — 生物安全柜

蒸汽供应管道 — 污水净化系统

机泵 — 生活污水

净化污水 — P4 实验室构造示意图

Filtered air exhaust   Breathing air system

Breathing air reservoir   Air handling unit

Exhaust fan   Outside air

Breathing air HEPA filter   Laboratory supply HEPA filter

Breathing hoses   APR window seal

Autoclave   Buffer corridor

APR inflatable seal door   Biosafety cabinets

Steam supply   Effluent decontamination system

Grinder pump   Sanitary waste

Decontaminated effluent

A Biosafety Level 4 Laboratory (BSL-4)

humans to humans, animals to humans, and animals to animals, namely microbes of BSL-3 (or pathogenic microorganisms categorized in Level 2, such as *Vibrio cholerae*, rabies virus, etc.).

BSL-4 laboratories: microorganisms handled at this level are those causing most severe diseases in humans and animals or those undiscovered or declared extinct in our country, namely microbes of BSL-4 (or pathogenic microorganisms categorized in Level 4, such as Ebola virus, Nipah virus, etc.).

As an old Chinese saying goes, "To do a good job, an artisan needs the best tools." The electron microscope enables the detailed study of viruses, with images obtained recording shapes and sizes of almost all known viruses, aiding in obtaining sufficient biological information. The PCR technique stores the nucleic acid sequence of various viruses isolated and detected, while biosafety laboratories provide platforms for protecting lab workers against virus infection, and humans have built and upgraded facilities of all biosafety levels.

As Chairman Mao wrote in his poem *Mountain Liupan*, "Today we hold the long cord in our hands, when shall we bind fast the Grey Dragon?"

CAR-T refers to Chimeric Antigen Receptor T-Cell Immunotherapy; CRISPR refers to Clustered Regularly Interspaced Short Palindromic Repeats, which is a sophisticated gene editing tool. Both tools can be used for precise localization and medical applications at a molecular cell level.

3. Cutting Edge

Active Immunity

Both the passive discovery of smallpox vaccine and the active development of rabies vaccine blazed a trail for the humankind's endeavor to combat viruses. Since then, preventive medical theory has been verified and applied in clinical practice, with the development of many viral vaccines and molecular biological techniques.

In 1963, Baruch Blumberg and Harvey Alter first discovered an abnormal antigen in the blood serum of two patients often receiving blood transfusions. The abnormal antigen could precipitate in the blood serum of an Australian Aborigine. In 1967, the antigen was identified specially associated with Hepatitis B virus (HBV). In 1970, the morphology of HBV particles was observed under an electron microscopy.

In 1971, the first Hepatitis B vaccine was approved for production. It was made from the hepatitis B surface antigen (HBsAg) that is purified from the plasma isolated and concentrated from asymptomatic carriers. In 1979, the HBsAg gene was cloned through molecular biology. In 1984, HBsAg in yeast was successfully developed into a vaccine to elicit protective immunity.

Natural virus-weakened vaccines, surface-antigen vaccines, and vaccines produced by genetic engineering all follow the law of the acquired immune system. With the stimulation of the viral antigen, the body can acquire an adaptive immune response, the process of which can be mainly divided into three stages: induction, response, and effect.

Dendritic cells and macrophages play important roles at the stage of induction. After phagocytosis of antigens such as bacteria and viruses, antigens processed can be identified by T cells and B cells and activate adaptive immune response of lymphocytes.

Stimulated by pathogenic agents at the stage of induction, B cells, with the assistance from helper T cells, can transform into plasma cells that can produce antibodies. The plasma cells can produce antibodies against pathogen-specific antigens and defend against pathogens through blood and humoral circulation in the body, the process of which is commonly referred to humoral immunity.

Stimulated by pathogenic agents at the stage of induction, T cells can release lymphocyte cytokines against specific pathogens by destroying antigen activity or enhancing the phagocytic and killing ability of macrophages. Lymphocyte cytokines can also activate T cells into cytotoxic T cells, which can exert immune effects and eliminate pathogens, the process of which is also known as cellular immunity.

The common way to determine whether a vaccine exerts protective effects on the body is through the antibody neutralization test, since antibodies in the blood circulatory system are easier to obtain when drawing

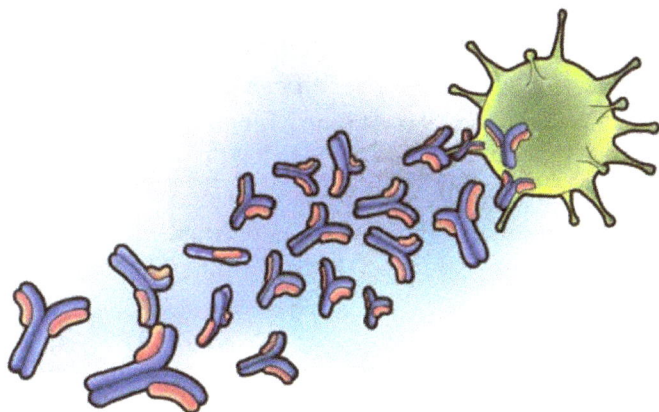

病毒中和抗体示意图

Antiviral Neutralizing Antibodies

blood. Humoral immunity and cellular immunity complement each other and jointly play the role in providing the immune response.

Memory cells maintain the production of antibodies after the adaptive immune response, whose duration determines the vaccine protection cycle. Therefore, the body can be protected for a long time or even acquire lifelong immunity after suffering from a disease or being inoculated with a specific vaccine.

Smallpox vaccination may induce a life-long immunity to smallpox. HBV vaccination gives protection for 3–10 years or even more than 20 years.

Therefore, vaccines indirectly fight against viruses by activating the body's immune system.

Antiviral Drugs

The general idea behind antiviral drug design is to directly fight against the virus itself. The anti-flu drug Tamiflu will be introduced in Section 3 of Chapter 8, and is a good example of an antiviral drug design. It is important to first clarify antibiotics are not antiviral drugs. Why? The answer will be given in Chapter 5.

There is a specific virus in the world. Humans have racked their brains to conquer it and even designed a series of antiviral drugs fighting against its every life cycle. To achieve higher efficiency of drugs, various drugs to combat this virus have to be combined for treatment, which is termed Highly Active Antiretroviral Therapy (HAART), or "cocktail therapy."

The virus in question is the human immunodeficiency virus (HIV), which leads to acquired immunodeficiency syndrome in those who are infected — it is also known as AIDS. Like life cycles of all the other viruses, cells attacked by HIV undergo the process of adsorption, replication in cells, and release of new viruses.

Round One

- HIV: on entering the body, the virus uses its "sugar coating," the membrane protein, to deceive CD4, the "monitor" on the surface of helper T cells. Then, the HIV gp41 protein acts as a "bridge" to break the cell membrane and fuses into the cell.
- HIV entry inhibitor — the virus fails to build the "bridge" to the cell when HIV entry inhibitor binds to HIV gp41 protein, which prevents HIV from fusing into the cell "wall."

Round Two

- HIV — Just like "a turtledove taking over the nest of a magpie," the virus starts to seize the time to make and assemble components by using raw materials from the cell.
- HIV uses its reverse transcriptase to convert the viral RNA to DNA by making use of the cell's nucleotides. HIV integrase integrates into the genome of the host cell's nucleus, synthesizing in parallel to cell replication.
- HIV reverse transcriptase inhibitor — Disguising as the nucleic acid raw material, the HIV reverse transcriptase inhibitor combines with HIV reverse transcriptase, hindering the synthesis of viral genetic material through termination of the "assembly line" caused by errors.
- HIV integrase inhibitor — By inhibiting integrase activity, the HIV integrase inhibitor blocks the integration of viral DNA into the cell genome.

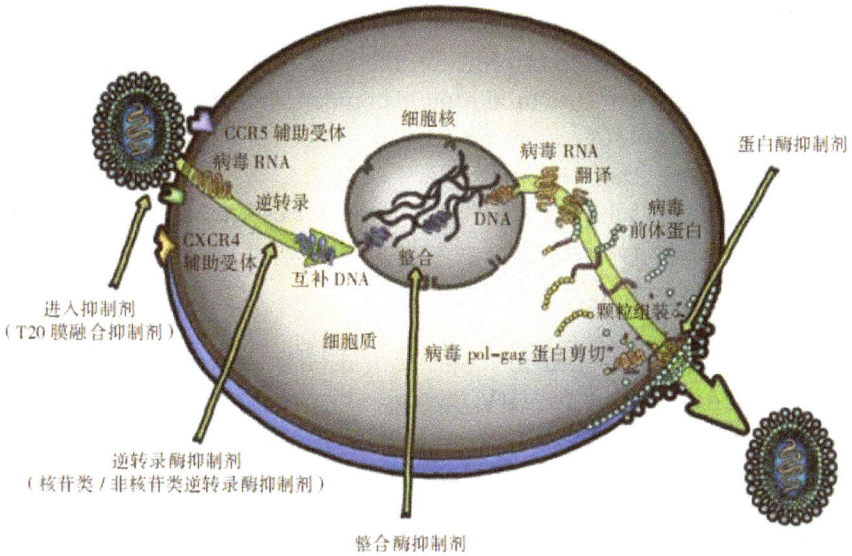

CCR5 辅助受体
病毒 RNA
逆转录
CXCR4 辅助受体
互补 DNA
进入抑制剂（T20 膜融合抑制剂）
逆转录酶抑制剂（核苷类／非核苷类逆转录酶抑制剂）
整合酶抑制剂
细胞核
DNA
整合
细胞质
病毒 pol-gag 蛋白剪切
病毒 RNA
翻译
病毒前体蛋白
颗粒组装
蛋白酶抑制剂

抗 HIV 药物：多回合持久较量

CCR5 Co-receptor

Viral RNA

Reverse transcription

CXCR4 Co-receptor

Entry inhibitors (T-20 fusion inhibitors)

Reverse transcriptase inhibitors

Nucleus

Complementary DNA

Integration

Cytoplasm

Integrase inhibitors

Viral RNA

Translation

Viral precursor protein

Particle Assembly

Viral gag-pol protein cleavage

Protease inhibitors

Anti-HIV drugs: a variable fighting with multiple rounds.

Round Three

- HIV — With the help of protease, the viral protein is assembled into the functional and structural protein component that is to be packaged together with RNA, releasing a large number of newborn HIV particles to infect other helper T cells.
- HIV protease inhibitor — With the protease function disrupted by HIV protease inhibitor, the precursor protein is prevented from the formation of viral "component."

Each drug is designed to target critical HIV reproductive cycles to inhibit or kill the virus for HIV therapy. "Cocktail therapy" is the most effective way to block AIDS though it fails to cure AIDS completely. Antiretroviral drugs can help HIV carriers and patients live a qualified life by effectively controlling and preventing the transmission of the virus.

Probably, this is destined to be a battle in the future.

CRISPR

In 1986, Diego Maradona won the FIFA World Cup for Argentina with his "Hand of God" goal.

In 1990, a fairy tale of love in a castle on a snowy and icy Christmas was clipped in *Edward Scissorhands*, a Hollywood fantasy film.

Thirty years later, the gene editing technology of CRISPR/Cas9, known as the "Hand of God" and "Magic Scissors," was listed as one of Science's Top 10 Breakthroughs of 2013 by *Science*. The rapid development of this technology led to a revolution in biomedical research and made it possible for us to "clip" diseases and "guard" health .

CRISPR/Cas9 system, an acquired immune defense mechanism evolved to resist the constant attack of viruses and plasmids, is an adaptive immune system in bacteria and archaea. Composed of clustered regularly interspaced short palindromic repeats (CRISPR) and CRISPR-associated (Cas) proteins, it can resist invasions of bacteria, viruses, or plasmids.

Plasmids are DNA molecules that replicate independently in such biological cells as bacteria and yeasts. As a gene carrier widely used in molecular biology, the plasmid can transfer the target gene into the cell to modify the original trait of the cell or produce target functional proteins, such as artificial insulin, genetically engineered hepatitis B vaccine, HIV inhibitors, etc.

The process is involved in reprogramming the plasmid, then transferring it into the cell, and finally knocking out or knocking in transformed recombinant genes. However, CRISPR/Cas9 is an unusual existence. Perhaps due to the long history of CRISPR/Cas9 system and the simple style of archaea, the guide RNA formed in the CRISPR system accurately "locates" the DNA molecule region of interest and then directs the Cas9 nuclease to "clip" the target DNA fragment for gene editing.

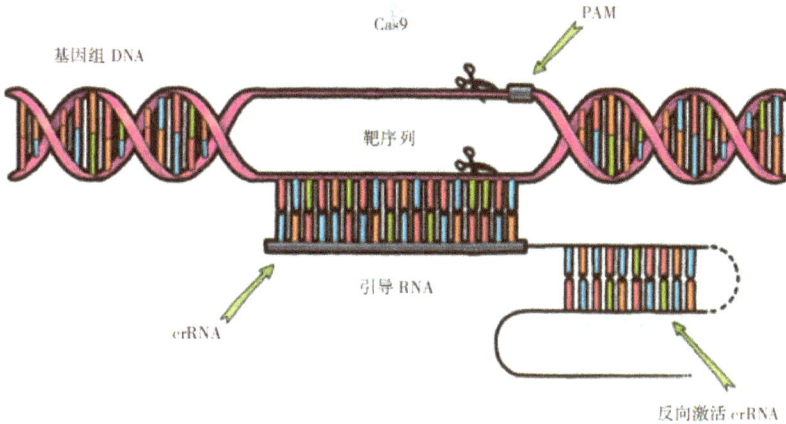

CRISPR/Cas9: 基因编辑之 "魔剪"

Genomic DNA   Cas9   PAM

Target Sequence

crRNA Guide RNA trans-activating crRNA

CRISPR/Cas9: "Magic Scissor" of Gene Editing

Genetic engineering follows the principle of "gene recombination→cell transformation→gene recombination," and sometimes multi-gene recombination and multi-cell transformation are required to achieve the target function, while CRISPR/Cas9 gene editing can obtain the target function simply by "gene localization→gene editing," just like the "magic scissor in God's hand."

In 2015, scientists in La Sierra University, California, USA, used the CRSPR/Cas9 technique to clip a specific DNA region of the HIV virus, inactivating 18%–72% of HIV in infected cells of the body. In 2016, this technique was used successfully in targeting a specific region of the HIV-1 DNA provirus, effectively and safely removing HIV from cultured human T cells. It is expected that these achievements will be applied to the clinical treatment of AIDS and have great potential for the treatment of viral infectious diseases and other diseases.

The CRISPR/Cas9 system, featuring powerful gene-editing function, is a significant discovery and creation in life science, which can be applied in many living organisms and scientific research fields, such as screening for functional genes and site-specific gene editing, drug target screening and validation, animal model construction, gene therapy of human diseases, etc.

Further development and improvement of the CRISPR/Cas9 system has led to its widespread applications in various research studies in life science, and it will have a bright future in human medicine despite occasionally selecting "off-target" genes.

God creates viruses and humans, and he also creates scissors.

CAR-T

When one first hears the term CAR-T, one might wonder whether it is a model T car. Let us name it "T cell car." However, the "T cell car" is not a new type of car but an innovative cellular immunotherapy. It is a remarkable "car" that carries a new life to the patient.

The world's first drug based on CAR-T cell therapy was approved by US Food and Drug Administration (FDA) in 2017. CAR-T is the abbreviation for chimeric antigen receptor T-cell therapy.

A large numbers of T cells act as "good guys" and "heroes" like doctors and policemen in our body. They are always patrolling in the blood. Whenever they detect such "bad guys" as mutated cells and cancer cells, they will immediately give a signal shot to call more cells for help in their rushing to the frontline to eliminate these "bad guys." Cancer will occur when "good guys" fail to recognize "bad guys" or eliminate them due to the weakened fighting force. In vitro, we can help to increase the activity of those weakened T cells and arm them with "heavy weapons," namely CAR-T.

The underlying principle of CAR-T is to eliminate cancer cells with the patient's own immune cells. It is a cell therapy and an immunotherapy approach rather than a drug. Compared to natural T cells, the modified ones can recognize a wider range of targets with the upgraded ability to identify tumor antigens, which has significant effectiveness on the treatment of acute leukemia and lymphoma.

CAR T-cell therapy generally involves the following steps:

- Step 1: Immune T cells are isolated from cancer patients, namely "reviewing troops";
- Step 2: The isolated immune T cells are modified through genetic engineering in vitro to obtain chimeric antigen receptor function which can recognize tumor cells and exert an effect on them. These T cells will become "superheroes" with "heavy weapons";
- Step 3: The CAR T cells are expanded by using a variety of culture systems to generate sufficient numbers for clinical therapy, namely "army expansion";
- Step 4: The CAR T cells which meet requirements of genetic engineering quality are infused back into patients according to the therapeutic dose, namely "fighting";
- Step 5: To maintain patients' health by relieving strong immune responses caused by the entry of CAR T cells into the body, namely "logistics."

In 2012, CAR-T therapy was first clinically tested in 30 patients with leukemia, who failed in the prior conventional chemotherapy and even bone marrow transplantation. Cancer cells completely disappeared in 27 of them after treatment and did not reoccur in 20 of them in the reexamination six months later. Particularly, some patients remained healthy six years later, among whom, Emily Whitehead, a beautiful and lively little girl, bravely enjoyed a cancer-free life of vitality after receiving CAR-T

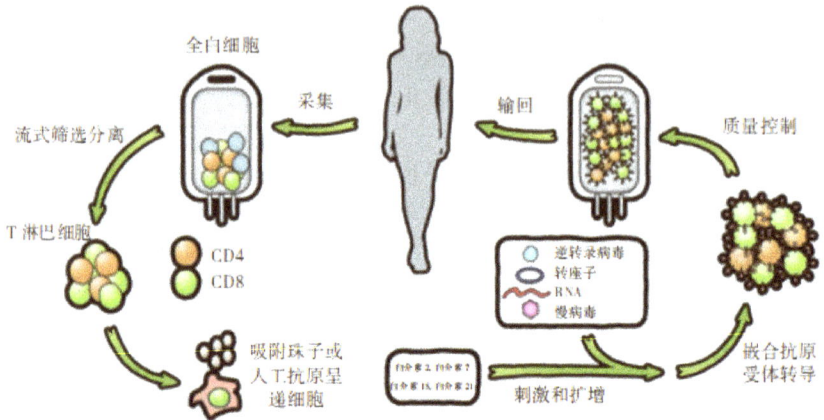

CAR-T 疗法示意图

Flow sorting column separation

T cells

Total white cells

CD4

CD8

Absorbed beads or artificial antigen-presenting cells

Pheresis

Return to patient

Retrovirus

Transposons

RNA

Lentivirus

Interleukin 2, Interleukin 7, Interleukin 15, Interleukin 21

Stimulation and expansion

Quality control

Chimeric antigen receptor transduction

CAR-T therapy

therapy experiment, inspiring the world to regard immunotherapy as a treatment of cancer.

CAR-T kills target cells by building specific chimeric antigen receptors that specifically recognize target antigens. It is also because of the "specific" cellular immunity mechanism that there are such corresponding clinical risks as cytokine storm. T cells effectively killing tumor cells will release a lot of cytokines, which will further activate intensive immune responses in the body, with the clinical symptom of inflammation. If this process is too intense, normal physiological functions of the body will be affected or even destroyed. The aftermath of the "storm" cannot be imagined once the disturbance is beyond the extent that the human body can tolerate.

Therefore, "logistics" is a critical step in CAR-T cell therapy. At the early development stage of CAR-T therapy, the patient receiving the therapy have a fever and even a coma. Fortunately, the timely rescue "comfort" cell "troops." Common symptoms include fever, rash, chills, hypotension, and even tumor lysis syndrome in severe cases. With greater clinical experience and scientific nursing guidance, the side effects of CAR-T therapy will be further reduced.

So far, the "T cell car" has been applied in clinical practice for only about several years. More time is required for testing its therapeutic effects. However, the proposal and application of this new cell therapy concept not only demonstrate the technological breakthrough of cell genetic engineering but also predict the upcoming of a new era of cell therapy in medicine.

Vaccines prevent diseases by infusing external "antigens" into the body to induce immune responses of immune cells in the body; while CAR-T plays the therapeutic role in the body by means of obtaining immune cells from the human body, arming them with the ability of recognizing and killing "antigens" in vitro, and infusing them back into body.

Thus, how about defining "antigen" as "virus"?

Who are the real foes that we face?

Chapter 5

To Catch a Cold

As noted in "Chill-heat Alternating Without Swelling" from the *Golden Mirror of Medicine: Knowledge and Skills of External Medicine in Verse* in Song Dynasty, "Chill-heat alternating is like cold or wind evil." Chen Hu, an imperial college student in Song Dynasty, created "Ganfeng Bo," i.e., notes for seeking leave because of "feeling wind evil." As recorded in *Collection of Anecdotes in Tea Aroma Room* in Qing Dynasty, "Gan Mao becomes an excuse used when officials asking for a leave."

1. Note for Seeking Leave in Song Dynasty

With regard to sneezing, there is a superstition that the number of times you sneeze has different meanings. One sneeze means someone misses you, two sneezes mean someone talks bad behind your back, and three sneezes mean that you catch a cold.

At this moment, I cannot help sneezing once.

What does the familiar term "to catch a cold" really mean?

All the following symptoms seem to be inextricably associated with catching a cold: sneezing, nasal congestion, rhinorrhea, tears, coughing, respiratory obstruction, hoarseness, headache, fever, cold, sore throat, pharyngitis, tracheitis, pneumonia, feeling uncomfortable, unwillingness to talk, feeling unwell, etc. Clinical symptoms caused by respiratory diseases can be collectively referred to as "cold."

The definition of "cold" in the dictionary is originated from Taixue, the Imperial Academy in feudal China.

Chen Wuze, a medical scientist in Song Dynasty, wrote *Sanyin Ji Yi Bingzheng Fang Lun* (*Sanyin Fang* for short) (*Treatise on Three Categories of Pathogenic Factors*), in which he identified three types of disease causes, namely internal cause, external cause, and non-endogenous, non-exogenous cause. External causes refer to such six pathogenic factors as wind, cold, summer heat, dampness, dryness, and heat, while internal causes refer to seven emotions, namely joy, anger, sorrow, thinking, sadness, fear, and surprise. He put forward the treatment methods by exploring pathogenesis and pathological mechanisms of different syndrome types according to clinical symptoms.

Chen Wuze, whose given name was Yan and courtesy name was Hang or Hexi Daoren, put forward the theories of "seven emotions and six sensory pleasures" and "integration of triple causes," which were popular to some extent due to remarks of *Sanyin Fang* in *Siku Quanshu Zongmu Tiyao* (*Annotated Catalog of the Complete Imperial Library*), which states "each treatment method is reasonable with elegant but concise words compared with those in redundant and vulgar words."

Guan Ge, the authoritative administrative body in Song Dynasty responsible for books and history compilation, comprises "Jixianyuan" (the administration for the collection of ancient books), "Mige" (the imperial library), "Longtuge" (the administration for the collection of royal books, pictures, and treasures), among others.

In Southern Song Dynasty, a shift work system was established in Guan Ge, according to which a member should be on night duty. However, it was a common practice for members on night duty to slip away at that time, the excuse for which, a norm used by generations of members, was recorded as "abdominal pain or discomfort and night-shift exempt in Guan Ge" in the duty register. As recorded in *Brush Talks from Dream Brook*, an extensive book written by the polymath Chinese scientist and statesman Shen Kuo in Song Dynasty:

> "One member should be arranged to be on duty in Guan Ge every night. If he slips away, Guan Ge will be unattended that night, which is called 'night-shift exempt.' The 'night-shift exempt' should not exceed four

consecutive days and there must be someone on night duty on the fifth day. It is a norm to write 'abdominal pain or discomfort and night-shift exempt' as an excuse on the register. Therefore, the night-duty register of Guan Ge is traditionally called 'abdominal discomfort register.'"

Taixue was the national university in ancient China and the highest institution of learning in the Imperial Court to train students and officials. Chen Hu, a "Taixuesheng" (or college student) in Song Dynasty, was compelled to be on night duty in Guan Ge. When he slipped away at night, he wrote "Gan Feng," meaning "feeling wind evil" in the register instead of using "abdominal pain or discomfort" as the excuse, which was the norm. "Gan" meant feeling, and "Feng" was one of the six external pathogenic causes. He recorded his creation in *Qijiu Xuwen* (*Anecdotes Collected by Chen Hu*):

"I, a Taixuesheng, wrote 'Gan Feng' in the register of the front porch to ask for a leave and get night-shift exempt. Thus, 'Haidu Li' (abdominal discomfort register) equals to 'Ganfeng Bo' (feeling wind register)."

"Ganfeng Bo" became an excuse used when officials asking for a leave in Qing Dynasty: I keep working hard for the official business though I have been ill for a long time; but now I have to ask for a sick leave for severe symptoms caused by the disease. As recorded in *Chaxiangshi Congchao* (*Collection of Anecdotes in Tea Aroma Room*) by Yu Yue, a scholar in Qing Dynasty, "Ganfeng Bo, originated from Song Dynasty, becomes an excuse used when officials asking for a leave today."

In this case, first, catching a cold is a state of illness rather than an illness. Second, catching a cold is directly associated with asking for a leave. It is not necessary for those registered in "Ganfeng Bo" to ask for a leave in the past. But now if you catch a cold and want to be absent from work, you are required to ask for a leave. Third, those who use catching a cold as an excuse to ask for a leave may not really get sick. Coincidentally, people worldwide seem to have the same understanding toward catching a cold, which can be heard from their daily expressions. "Zhao Liang" (catching a chill) is a Chinese phrase to indicate "catching a cold," which is often used by Chinese people with a tone of grief and sorrow in their daily conversations. Similarly, "to catch a cold" is also an English expression, with the literal meaning of "Zhao Liang" in Chinese, followed by British people's complaint about "bad weather."

Sometimes, the weather is unpredictable, and cold weather does make people catch a chill and weaken their immunity. However, something dangerous lurking in the cold weather is waiting for the opportunity to invade the body... it is the real cause of catching a cold, although humans cannot see it directly with their eyes.

Today, those attacked by common cold, dragging their tired bodies to hospitals, are often informed that they may have either bacterial or viral cold. Particularly in hot weather, doctors perhaps will not tell you that the cause is "catching a chill." Measures should be taken to fight the culprit that causes cold. Thus, let us get to know "bad guys" in the air. In fact, these invisible microbes have been hiding in our environment all the time.

Bacteria and viruses, we have known you for a very short time, but you have known our world very well: you are indeed "bad boys" hiding in the air!

Common cold in humans can be divided into bacterial cold and viral cold. Pathogenic agents of the former are bacteria such as *Diplococcus pneumoniae*, *Streptococcus*, *Staphylococcus aureus*, and *Bacillus influenzae*. Antibiotic drugs can be used to fight these pathogenic bacteria.

2. Bacterial Cold

Reviewing the "flavor of French broth," let us go back to the European continent at the end of the 19th century, when two giants of science put forward the theory of microbial pathogenesis. Louis Pasteur, a French microbiologist, discovered that bacteria could cause diseases when studying microbial fermentation and anthrax. In his study of tuberculosis and anthrax bacillus, Robert Koch, a German bacteriologist, put forward "Koch's Postulates," the classic guiding principle of microbial discovery.

Koch's Postulates, also known as criteria for disease causation, are often used to identify the causative agent of an infectious disease, which include:

(1) bacteria must be present in every case of the disease, and be absent in the healthy body;

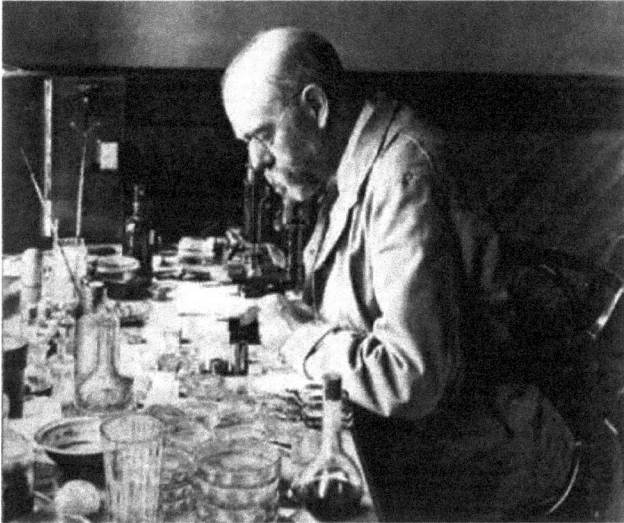

罗伯特·科赫在实验室

Robert Koch in the Laboratory.

(2) bacteria must be isolated from the host with the disease and grown in pure culture;

(3) specific disease must be reproduced when a pure culture of bacteria is inoculated into a healthy susceptible host;

(4) bacteria must be recoverable from the experimentally infected host.

If the above four criteria are fulfilled, the bacteria can be identified as pathogenic agents.

"Cold" bacteria, which cause such severe respiratory diseases as pneumonia, include *Staphylococcus aureus*, *Streptococcus*, and *Mycobacterium tuberculosis*, among others. The typical *Staphylococcus aureus*, around 0.8 microns in diameter, is cocci-shaped. It is observed to be arranged in clusters that are described as "grape-like" under a microscope and is often golden or yellow after microbial staining. *Streptococcus*, 0.5–1 micron in diameter, is generally cocci or oval-shaped, most of which are arranged in chains. *Streptococcus*, named for its chain shape, consists of at least 5–10 bacteria or 20–30 bacteria at maximum. *Mycobacterium tuberculosis*, the pathogenic bacterium causing tuberculosis, is a slightly curved, rod-shaped bacilli, with 1–4 microns in length and around 0.4 microns in diameter. Tuberculosis continues to be a major infectious disease severely threatening public health.

World War II began in the Eurasia continent and spread to the rest of the world, from the land to the ocean, and from the ocean to the sky. As the largest world war in human history, over 2 billion people from 61 countries and regions were involved, and there were more than 90 million military and civilian casualties in the theater of war covering 22 million square kilometers. The main Axis powers were Germany's Third Reich, Fascist Italy, and Imperial Japan, while Allied powers included the US, the Soviet Union, Britain, France, and China, among others. Soldiers on the battlefield usually died of such physical battle-related injuries as vital organ damage. For those wounded in the battle, invisible infections such as festering and inflammation of wounds would lead to disabilities or further casualties. Without prompt control of infections, their tissues and organs would further deteriorate. In severe cases, they cannot survive if their body functions were destroyed.

Following the clouds of artillery fire came the shadow of airborne pathogens, which caused invisible infections: tens of thousands of soldiers died of physical battle-related injuries every day. More terribly, there were soldiers dying from infected wounds due to lack of effective antibiotic drugs.

The British scientist Alexander Fleming, a military physician in World War I, treated wounded soldiers and studied their infected wounds and the effect of immunotherapy. He discovered that penicillium can produce a substance repressing *Staphylococcus* growth in an experiment. He named the substance Penicillin.

After the outbreak of World War II, Howard Florey, an Australian scientist, successfully cured an infected small animal by administering purified penicillin on it. He further attempted to inject the purified penicillin to treat infected humans, among whom, more penicillin doses are required for the treatment of adults.

Howard Florey traveled to the US to work with Hermann Muller. They isolated the mold which yielded 200 times the amount of penicillin extract and even tens of thousands of times with the X-ray-radiation–induced engineered bacteria. The US officially introduced penicillin in 1943, a highly effective anti-infection drug. The large-scale production of penicillin in 1944 helped heal wounded soldiers who had bacterial infection. Penicillin, with the prestige of "equivalent of 20 divisions of troops," greatly increases the life expectancy of humans.

Streptomycin, the second antibiotic after penicillin, was isolated from *Streptomyces* by an American scientist Selman Waksman in 1943. It is an antibiotic specific to *Mycobacterium tuberculosis*, changing the history of incurable tuberculosis from then on.

They further isolated over 20 antibacterial substances from soil microbes and named them "antibiotics," which refer to metabolites with anti-pathogenic activity produced by microbes or higher plants and animals.

Cephalosporin was first discovered from the beach soil in Sardinia in 1948. Cephalosporin C was isolated in 1955. Semi-synthetic cephalosporins were developed in the 1960s. Subsequently, four generations of cephalosporins were developed one after another. At present, the fifth generation of cephalosporin is available.

How do antibiotics work as the "weapon" to protect human health in the "battlefield" against bacteria? The essential structures of bacteria are cell walls, membranes, cytoplasm, and nucleoli. The common components of human cells contain cell membranes, cytoplasm, organelles, and nucleus. Human cells do not have cell walls, while cell walls are essential components of bacterial cells. With similar molecular structures to the cell wall, penicillin can inhibit cell wall synthesis of bacteria by binding to transpeptidase and blocking mucin synthesis of the cell wall, analogous to "replacing beams with rotten timbers." Failing to form complete cell walls, bacteria will be "broken into pieces" and die of cell function destruction.

Similar to the antibacterial mechanism of penicillin, cephalosporins inhibit the synthesis of bacterial cell walls, alters cell membrane permeability, and cause bacterial cell lysis or prevent bacteria from reproducing themselves by releasing autolysin. The advent of antibiotics makes it possible to conquer *Staphylococcus* infections, pneumonia, and tuberculosis.

As the Chinese idiom goes, "virtue is one foot tall, the devil ten feet." Due to antibiotics abuse and other reasons, pathogenic bacteria gradually realize though they are restrained by a certain antibiotic, and therefore develop antimicrobial resistance (AMR) via evolutionary mutation to

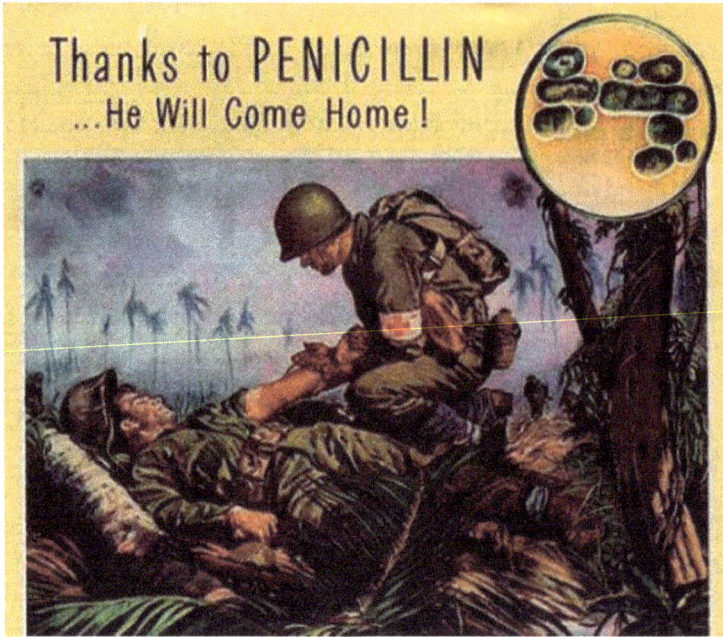

第二次世界大战期间海报

A Poster in World War II

avoid damage to their functions if antibiotics are repeatedly used to fight them.

Microbes were the first life on earth. Single-celled organisms such as bacteria, long before the advent of humans, actively adapted to and even modified the surrounding environment to survive under different conditions in the evolutionary process spanning a hundred millions years. Only a few bacteria survive in the battle with antibiotics. However, with the weakened fighting capacity, drug-resistant bacteria cannot escape when the body's immune system sweeps the surviving ones in the battlefield.

Antibiotic abuse by humans creates opportunities for pathogenic bacteria to become resistant and render antibiotics useless. If antibiotics cannot be used at the right dose or target specific bacteria, surviving drug-resistant bacteria will accumulate in the body. The repeated use of antibiotics for the treatment of infections will increase bacterial resistance, reduce the effectiveness of antibiotics, and even lead to no effective drugs available for treatment.

So far, penicillin series and cephalosporin series have developed antibiotics of 2.0/3.0 and other upgraded versions. With the development of different research levels in life science and breakthroughs of cross-integration of different biotechnologies, more advanced antibacterial drugs will be developed and synthesized through more sophisticated determination of pathogenic bacteria to produce antibiotics at different levels.

It is humans themselves who are competitors in this wholly new race.

Viral cold is caused by such viruses as rhinoviruses, adenoviruses, coronaviruses, and syncytial viruses. People infected with these viruses usually recover through their own immunity. After recognizing and fighting against viruses, immune cells produce neutralizing antibodies and evolve into killer cells to build up the systemic defense line and keep the body healthy.

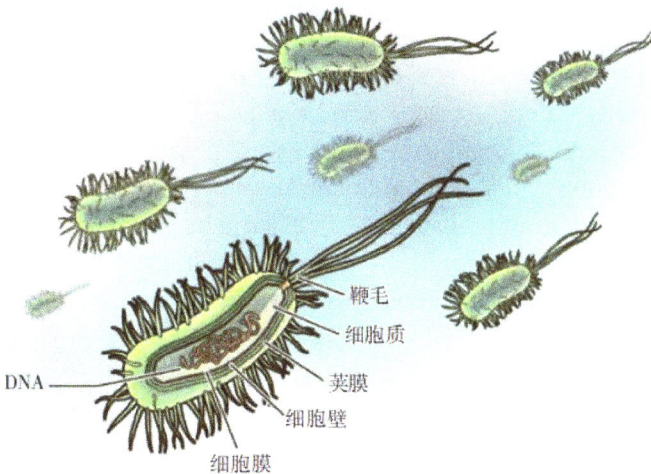

细菌结构形态示意图

Bacterial Structure and Morphology

3. Viral Cold

People will get common cold when bacteria "commit crime" in the body together with their accomplices, "malicious" viruses, on the "crime scene."

Rhinovirus, the main pathogenic agent causing common cold, was isolated by scientists from cultured specimens obtained in patients with respiratory infections. So far, more than 120 rhinoviruses have been identified. As main pathogenic agents of acute respiratory diseases, rhinoviruses are responsible for nearly half the numbers of acute respiratory infections. Rhinoviruses are active throughout the year. Spreading by airborne droplets or direct contact, they always cause such upper respiratory infections as common cold in adults and bronchitis or bronchopneumonia in children and babies or patients with chronic respiratory diseases.

Adenovirus can cause such respiratory infections as cough, nasal obstruction, and pharyngitis. More than 100 types have been discovered since it was isolated from human adenoids in 1953, of which 52 human adenoviruses are known to infect such organs as respiratory tract, gastrointestinal tract, urethra, and liver. Adenoviruses are most active in winter. They are mainly transmitted through respiratory tract or contact via respiratory tract droplets and eye secretions or through digestive tract to cause intestinal infections, acute febrile pharyngitis, conjunctivitis, acute respiratory diseases, Legionnaires' disease, children's pneumonia, etc.

Coronaviruses, first isolated in chickens in 1937, primarily infect the respiratory systems of humans. The first strain of human coronavirus was isolated in 1965, with prominent spikes protruding from its outer membrane. It was the SARS coronavirus that caused the global outbreak of severe acute respiratory syndrome (SARS) in 2002. In 2012, the novel MERS coronavirus was found to be responsible for Middle East Respiratory Syndrome (MERS) in Saudi Arabia. Coronavirus, with its peak infections in autumn, winter, and early spring, is transmitted via respiratory secretions, contact, and airborne droplets. As one of major pathogenic agents of common cold in adults, coronaviruses can cause upper respiratory tract infections in children and severe acute respiratory syndrome in humans.

Respiratory syncytial virus (RSV) is the most common pathogenic agent of viral pneumonia in children and infants. It can cause interstitial pneumonia and bronchiolitis, which can be infected by airborne droplets and close contact. Syncytial virus pneumonia and bronchiolitis, with similar symptoms to mild influenza viral pneumonia, were prevalent in the population in recent years. RSV is highly contagious in winter, spring, and summer, depending on different regions. Children and adults with upper respiratory tract infections are more likely to be infected by syncytial virus.

Let us take an example to explain how human body infected with viruses uses its own immune system to eradicate and defeat them.

Adenovirus is a non-enveloped and icosahedral viral particle that is 70–90 nanometers in diameter. The protein shell, composed of 252 capsomeres, contains linear double-stranded DNA molecules with the length of 26–48 kilobase pairs. The human body can develop effective immunity to an adenovirus infection. Vaccines are usually developed from attenuated pathogens or genetically engineered pathogen antigens to induce the immune system to produce protective neutralizing antibodies of specific pathogens. Therefore, there are two essential requirements for vaccine development: safety to the body and immune response triggered in the body.

Adenovirus itself is a kind of exogenous pathogen causing respiratory infectious diseases in humans. After being infected with viruses, the body's immune system often activates protective mechanisms to eradicate natural live viruses and produce immunity to these viruses through humoral and cellular immune response. Meanwhile, with the help of memory cells, this immunity will produce protective neutralizing antibodies in the body. Different adenovirus serotypes can produce disparate antibodies. Thus, there are many protective antibodies to different adenoviruses in a healthy body.

Due to the various virus types and unnecessary treatment based on the specific virus type, it is generally unnecessary to perform an etiology examination when contracting such common viral cold symptoms as upper respiratory tract infections, including nasal cavity, pharynx or larynx acute inflammation. Diagnosis of such infections can be made based on patients' medical history and epidemiological clinical symptoms, together with peripheral blood and chest imaging examination results. Therefore, such diseases can be treated by good rest, strengthening the constitution, reducing heat and pains, reliving symptoms, etc.

The common cold is usually a mild, self-limiting illness lasting for only a few days, and therefore has an excellent prognosis. From the "Ganfeng Bo" in Song Dynasty to "asking for a leave due to catching a cold" in Qing Dynasty, common cold is often used to ask for a leave, which is indeed a very reasonable excuse. If the excuse of asking for a leave is "severe typhoid fever," I'm afraid you will have no choice but to stay at home and lie in bed for at least 10–15 days even if the imperial physician is not required to verify the truth of the excuse.

It is because we know the "weakness" of bacterial cell walls and have the "defense" ability endowed by our immune cells that we can use antibiotics and our own immune system to prevent and fight the common cold caused by bacteria and viruses. However, if enemies disguise their weaknesses and improve their weapons, what can we do?

Is it possible for us to encounter more ferocious enemies?

Chapter 6

The Devil

Influenza viruses can cause flu in humans, leading to fever, body aches, obvious fatigue, or acute respiratory symptoms. Flu season always occurs in winter and spring. It is most likely to result in a pandemic since it is highly contagious and spreads quickly. It can cause severe syndrome of pneumonia or even death.

1. Influenza Viruses

In 1658, there were 60,000 deaths from the flu in the Venice, Italy. The unusually fierce flu spread to the UK and throughout the European continent. At that time, people believed that it was God's punishment or bad luck brought by devils in astrology that caused the flu outbreak. Therefore, the disease was named "influenza," similar to "influence" in Italian, which consisted of the affixes "in" + "flu" + "enza," meaning "introduce" + "prevalent" + "disease," namely prevalent diseases in human bodies. It was later particularly referred as flu.

- From 1742 to 1743, influenza caused diseases in 90% of population in Eastern Europe;
- In 1837, there was a severe flu outbreak in Europe, leading to the flu-related death rate exceeding the birth rate in Berlin and all public activities suspended in Barcelona;

- From 1889 to 1894, the flu outbreak in Western Europe killed around one million people around the world;
- In 1918, it was estimated that over 100 million people died from the global flu pandemic;
- In 1957, the Asian flu led to the death of an estimated two million people;
- In 1968, the flu spread from Hong Kong, China, and was transmitted to Europe and the US, leading to 30,000 deaths in the US;
- In 1977, Russian flu began in the Soviet Union;
- In 1999, there was a simultaneous flu outbreak in Asia, Europe, and the Americas, which developed into a severe flu in France;
- In 2009, the flu outbreak in the Americas killed about 20,000 people worldwide.

Influenza, or flu, is an acute respiratory tract infectious disease caused by flu viruses, which can spread rapidly via air droplets, person-to-person contact, or person-to-object contact.

Flu viruses are sensitive to heat, ultraviolet light, dryness, and most chemical disinfectants. It has been shown that flu viruses will lose their ability to infect within 30 minutes in an acidic environment with a pH of 2, or in a heated environment of 56 degree centigrade, or in a 70% alcohol solution, and they will be completely inactivated within 15 seconds in the iodophor solution (5 g/L).

Transmitted via droplets or aerosols in the air, flu viruses invade the body's respiratory tract mucous membrane, penetrate the mucus layer on the surface of respiratory tract, enter into such host cells as surface epithelial cells, and rapidly replicate themselves in host cells. It usually takes six hours for the infected cells to release a new generation of virions. Meanwhile, the production of protein toxins during the virus replication facilitates this cycle and increases the invasion speed.

There are about 300 million alveoli bounded by a surface of around 100 square meters in each human lung for the gas exchange between human blood and inhaled air with the ventilation rate of 6 L/min. at rest, during which, viruses and other foreign particles enter the lung.

Larger particles will be deposited in the upper respiratory tract, while smaller ones cannot be absorbed. Only those with diameters of

1–4 microns can enter trachea and alveoli. Some "enemy agent" molecules, flu virus aerosols, with the size between 1–4 microns in diameter, can launch sneak raids to the trachea and alveoli.

The complex cytopathic effect occurs after the invasion of viruses, which will lead to host cell damage or apoptosis as host cell proteins decrease. Normal cell apoptosis is the physiological and metabolic activity in humans, while the cell apoptosis caused by viruses will destroy functions of infected cells and even result in pathological changes of tissues and organs or organ failures and even death in severe cases.

The human host cells infected with flu virus are mainly in the respiratory mucus layer, digestive tract, endodermis, and myocardium, as well as brain. There are millions of viral particles in nasal secretions per milliliter, suggesting that aerosol per microliter contains over 1,000 flu virus particles. In general cases, it takes only 100 to 1,000 viral particles to make humans sick. Thus, again, "It is always good to get a mask."

Today, humans living in different continents are no longer separated by oceans or great mountains. We can go anywhere in the world by air in less than three days. Within the same day, you can experience a summer day in the south while I am in a winter night in the north. It takes less than six hours for viruses to complete the replication cycle in host cells and release themselves from the body to the environment. In most cases, the incubation period of flu is 2–4 days but can range from 1–7 days.

All these point to the fact that flu is a global issue.

Influenza viruses have two major surface glycoproteins, hemagglutinin (HA) and neuraminidase (NA), which are embedded in membrane envelopes. On average, 500 HA spikes and 100 NA spikes are present on the surface of a typical influenza virus. Influenza A viruses are classified into subtypes based on antigenic properties of their HA and NA, such as H1N1.

2. Influenza Families

Depending on different infected hosts, flu viruses can be classified into human influenza viruses, swine influenza viruses, equine influenza viruses, and avian influenza viruses. They can also be divided into the following four subtypes based on their antigenic properties of ribonucleoproteins:

- Influenza A Virus, or Influenza Type A Virus;
- Influenza B Virus, or Influenza Type B Virus;
- Influenza C Virus, or Influenza Type C Virus;
- Influenza D Virus, or Influenza Type D Virus.

Isolated from pigs in 1931 and from humans in 1933, influenza A virus, the main pathogen of human influenza, is prone to mutate and can infect humans and many different animals. Influenza B virus, which was isolated in 1940, can cause seasonal and regional infections of humans. Influenza C virus, which was isolated in 1947, can cause upper respiratory infections in humans. Influenza D virus was isolated in 2011 and officially named in 2016. It primarily infects cattle and pigs, with no human infection cases reported so far.

The "Four Heavenly Kings" have made their debut now. You may be confused since you are convinced that all viruses should be named as "HxNy." As a matter of fact, influenza A viruses are classified into subtypes based on antigenic differences of structural proteins hemagglutinin (HA) and neuraminidase (NA) embedded in their surfaces. So far, 18 HA subtypes and 11 NA subtypes have been identified. Among the known subtypes, HA (H17/18) and NA (N10/11) have been found in bats' genes. However, no virus has been isolated from them and no evidence has shown these gene fragments can recombine with other influenza A viruses.

There are two Groups in 18 HA subtypes of influenza A virus. Group 1 subtypes are H1, H2, H5, H6, H8, H9, H11, H12, H13, H16, H17, and H18 and Group 2 subtypes are H3, H4, H7, H10, H14, and H15.

WHO's naming conventions for various influenza viruses are as follows:

- The virus type (e.g., A, B, C, D);
- For human-origin viruses, no host of origin designation is given; for animal-origin viruses, the host of origin designation is given;
- Geographical origin where the flu virus was isolated (e.g., Yamagata and Victoria);
- Laboratory strain number;

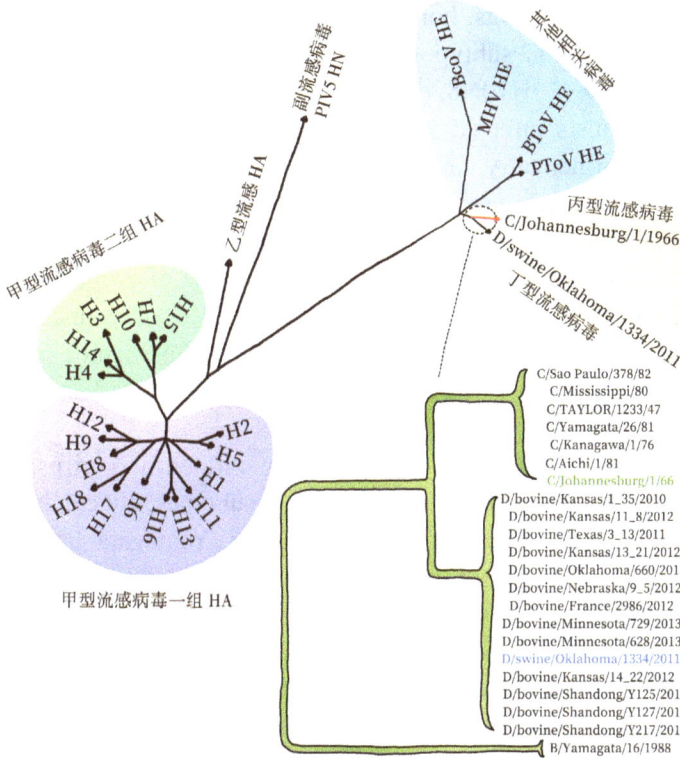

Group I influenza A HA
Group II influenza A HA
Influenza B virus
Parainfluenza virus PIV5 HN
Other related viruses
Influenza C virus
Influenza D virus
Influenza virus types: A, B, C and D

- Year of virus isolation;
- For avian influenza viruses, HA and NA subtypes should be designated.

Influenza A virus can infect humans, mammals, and birds. H1N1, H2N2, and H3N2 subtypes mainly infect humans, while other subtypes primarily infect birds, pigs, horses, and aquatic mammals. Among avian flu viruses, there are 12 subtypes infecting humans, such as H5N1, H7N1, H7N2, H7N9, H9N2, H10N8, etc.

In animal hosts infected with influenza A virus, birds can be only infected with influenza A virus. So far, 16 HA subtypes and 9 NA subtypes of avian influenza viruses have been isolated, including typical ones such as H5N2 and H7N7; influenza virus subtypes H17, H18, N10, and N11 were mainly isolated in bats; the main subtype of swine flu virus is H1N1; H7N7 and H3N8 are the main known subtypes of equine influenza virus; influenza virus subtypes of H1N1, H3N2, H3N8, and H5N1 were isolated in dogs; besides, cats and mice can also be infected and carry flu viruses.

Influenza B viruses, less prevalent than influenza A virus, mainly spread in humans. They are not classified into subtypes, but can be broken into three lineages, including the Lee lineage, Yamagata lineage, and Victoria lineage. Influenza C viruses, isolated from pigs, do not usually infect humans. But rare human infections have occurred. Influenza D viruses were recently discovered and isolated from animals.

Therefore, it can be seen that among "Four Heavenly Kings," influenza A viruses are the "Central Army" as well as "elite division" of HA and NA subtypes: H1N1, H2N2, and H3N3.

H1N1 Flu Virus

H1N1 flu virus, one of the most common influenza viruses to infect humans, can also infect birds and pigs. It has been found that pigs are intermediate hosts (or reservoir hosts) of human influenza viruses and avian influenza viruses as well as the vital source of virus genetic recombination ("mixer").

As the cause of global pandemic in 1918, H1N1 broke out in North America and spread across the world in 2009, with around 20,000 people from 213 countries killed. WHO raised the worldwide pandemic alert level to phase 6, the highest alert level. It seemed that "Spanish Lady" returned.

The most remarkable feature of H1N1 infection is the sudden outbreak and rapid spread. The H1N1 pandemic in 2009 spread to 23 countries and regions on four continents in around 10 days. Confirmed deaths were mainly young people aged 25 to 45 years. Severe cases and deaths also occurred. Patients had a high recessive infection rate in the incubation period after infection. H1N1 remains prevalent in humans every year.

H2N2 Flu Virus

Within 40 years after the 1918 pandemic, the flu became less virulent and only occurred in certain regions. In 1957, the influenza pandemic, known as Asian flu, swept through the world. The first cases were reported in Guizhou and Yunnan Provinces in China in February to April. Then Asian flu affected other provinces and Hong Kong and Taiwan in China. In May, Singapore and Japan also experienced an outbreak of the flu. In June, the flu spread to Southwest Asia, Oceania, Europe, and North America. From July to August, Asian flu broke out in many parts of the world, including Africa, South America, the Pacific Islands, and the Caribbean.

The influenza virus attacking humans was H2N2 subtype, with humans and birds as its main hosts. The Asian flu outbreak was featured by high morbidity and mortality. It has been shown that Asian flu, with the peak incidence rate of over 50%, mainly infected people aged 5 to 19years, and killed millions of people.

Typical clinical symptoms caused by H2N2 influenza virus are respiratory diseases and the most common complication leading to death is viral pneumonia. The H2N2 flu virus did not infect humans again after the "Asian flu" outbreak, while it remains to be isolated from poultry and wild birds, making it possible to spread to humans again.

H3N2 Flu Virus

The flu was also named "Hong Kong flu" since Hong Kong, China, was the epicenter of the outbreak. In 1968, H3N2 flu outbreak started in southern China and Hong Kong, China, spread to Southeast Asia and gradually became the third global pandemic. In July, it spread from Hong Kong, China, to Singapore, Thailand, Japan, India, and Australia. In autumn, it reached Europe and attacked the Americas at the end of the year; it invaded South America and South Africa in 1969; the second flu peak occurred in 1970, with the virus prevailing in the southern summer and northern winter. The flu killed 34,000 people in the US and 750,000 people worldwide.

H3N2, with humans as its main hosts, remains to be the main subtype infecting humans. It usually causes acute respiratory infectious disease, pneumonia, and respiratory failure in severe cases and even death; this subtype, featuring rapid onset and high incidence, is highly contagious and widely prevalent. People at all ages are susceptible to this virus. Particularly the elderly, children, and those physically weak are more likely to get sick after being exposed to the virus. The asymptomatic people are the main source of infection.

The virus can be transmitted via respiratory tracts of different animals. The risk of genetic recombination is increased due to various hosts of H3N2 influenza virus, such as pigs, birds, and humans. Besides, symptoms of people infected with the virus are similar to those of the common flu. Therefore, the virus is also a dangerous enemy for humans to watch out.

All these indicate that influenza is a host-and-virus issue.

The invisible flu virus, the prime culprit causing influenza, can be transmitted via air droplets or contact. Virus particles are usually spherical in shape and 80–120 nanometers in diameter. A virion consists

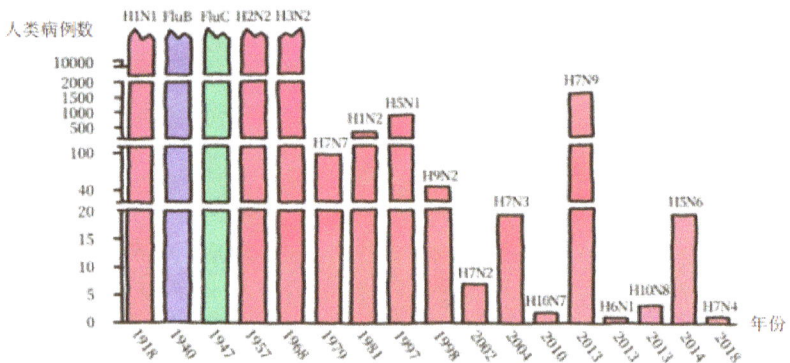

人感染流感病毒年份表

Human Infection Cases: Year and Infection Cases with Influenza Viruses in 100 Years.

of envelope, matrix protein, and nucleic core containing single-stranded RNA genetic material.

3. Influenza Virions

Nucleic Core

The flu virus core contains the genetic material and viral proteinase necessary for the replication of genetic information.

The genetic material of flu virus is single-stranded RNA (ss-RNA), which binds to nuclear protein and winds up to the highly dense Ribonucleoprotein Complex (RNP). Besides, there are RNA polymerases responsible for RNA transcription.

Genomes of influenza A virus and influenza B virus are composed of eight RNA gene segments. Segment 1, segment 2, and segment 3 encode for the RNA polymerase; segment 4 encodes for HA; segment 5 encodes for nucleocapsid protein; segment 6 encodes for NA; segment 7 encodes for matrix protein; and segment 8 encodes for a nonstructural protein splicing RNA functions. Genomes of influenza C virus and influenza D virus consists of seven RNA gene segments, among which HA and NA are encoded by the same segment.

Nucleocapsid protein, the structural protein encoded by segment 5, is responsible for the transcription and replication of viral genomes and the formation of nucleocapsid of viruses. As the most conservative one, the nucleoprotein can serve as the classification standard of virus subtypes based on its specific antigens.

Influenza virus polymerase is composed of three proteins encoded by three RNA segments: PA, PB1, and PB2, performing the function of replicase genes. Amino acids in these three proteins are nucleophilic, allowing them to enter the nucleus and synthesize viral genetic information in cells.

Matrix Protein

Matrix Protein (M) is the shell skeleton of the virus. It includes structural protein (M1) and membrane protein (M2). Tightly binding to the outermost

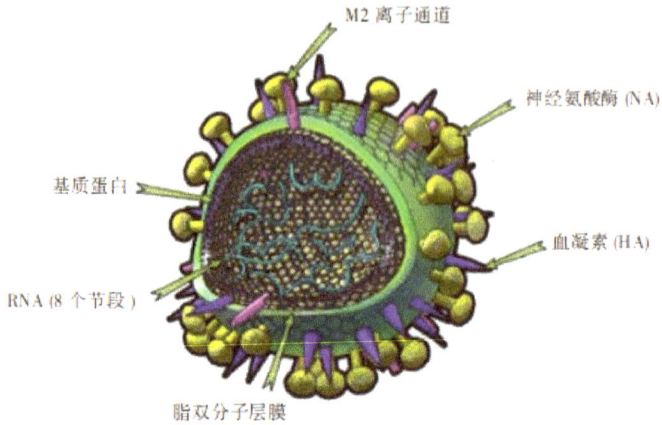

M2 离子通道
神经氨酸酶 (NA)
基质蛋白
血凝素 (HA)
RNA (8 个节段)
脂双分子层膜

流感病毒结构模型图

Matrix protein. RNA (8 segments)
Lipid bilayer membrane
Hemagglutinin (HA)
Neuraminidase (NA)
M2 ion channel
Influenza Virus Structure

membrane of virus, M1 is responsible for protecting the core of the virus and maintaining its spatial structure. M2 can serve as an ion channel and regulate pH values.

After flu viruses replicate themselves in host cells, formed viral nucleocapsids can recognize structural proteins on the inner walls of host cell membranes and combine with them on host cell membranes to produce virions, which can be protruded and released in the form of buds.

Envelope

The influenza virus envelope is a layer of phospholipid bilayer enclosing matrix protein, which is derived from the host cell membrane. The mature influenza virus, which is released from the infected host cell, wraps the cell membrane around virion and then leaves the infected cell to attack another host cell.

In addition to phospholipid molecules, there are two very important glycoproteins in the envelope: HA and NA. The antigenicity of the influenza virus nucleoprotein can be used to determine influenza types, and HA and NA antigenicity can be used to determine influenza virus subtypes.

HA

The HA of the influenza virus is columnar and can bind to receptors on the surface of red blood cells of humans and animals such as birds and guinea pigs and cause blood clots. After HA proteolysis, it is divided into two parts: light chain and heavy chain. The latter can be combined with the sialic acid receptors on the host cell membrane. The former can assist the fusion of the viral envelope and the host cell membrane. HA plays an important role in the introduction of virus into host cells. HA is immunogenic and anti-HA antibodies neutralize influenza viruses, which can be designed as important components of antiviral vaccines.

NA

The NA of the influenza virus is a mushroom-shaped tetramer of identical subunits, with sialic acid hydrolysis activity. When a mature influenza virus is ready to leave the host cell, the HA on the virus surface still binds the virus to the sialic acid receptor on the host cell membrane. To be successfully released from the infected host cell and continue to infect another one, the connection between the virus and infected host cell should be cut off with the help of NA via sialic acid hydrolysis. Therefore, NA becomes the target of influenza therapy, and anti-influenza drugs can be designed according to this protease.

Influenza viruses have been fully armed and ready to attack humans. What kind of time and space storm happened in the microcosm within six hours?

Influenza viruses bind to cellular glycoproteins or sialic acids in the glycolipid via HA, so that flu viruses can bind to the surface of host cells. Influenza viruses can infect many types of cells in the body since saccharide sialic acids are present on different cells in the body and HA is able to bind to sialic acids.

When the virus is attached to the host cell, the cell membrane protein receptor will mediate the endocytosis of the virus, facilitating the fusion between virus and the endocyte to form the phagocyte. The viral substance will be released as the pH value in the phagocytosis gradually decreases. When the pH value drops to a certain level, M2 will be activated to terminate the decline of pH value and enable HA to function.

HA fuses with the endosomal membrane and releases the ribonucleoprotein complex into the cytoplasm. Proteins in virions are dissociated and ribonucleoprotein complexes are released and removed from viruses. The whole process only lasts 20–30 minutes.

Ribonucleoprotein complexes are transported to the nucleus, where polymerase binds to viral RNA. The RNA transcripts exist in the form of mRNA with restricted binding to nucleoproteins. mRNA transcripts and nucleoproteins are then transported to the cytoplasm for the synthesis of viral proteins on ribosomes.

Some newly synthesized viral proteins are transported to the nucleus, where they form ribonucleoprotein complexes by binding to viral RNA. Other newly synthesized viral proteins are processed in the endoplasmic reticulum and the Golgi apparatus where glycosylation occurs. These modified viral proteins are transported to the cell membrane. When the concentration is high enough, they aggregate and condense to produce new virus particles. Finally, the particle is extruded from the membrane and will then be liberated by the NA activity.

From the entry of a host cell to the production of a new virion, the flu virus performs wonderful life moments in its play of "out of" and "into" human cells on its way to survive.

The truth of flu virus nature has been revealed to us. The following questions in both previous and current chapters remain to be addressed:

Question one: why adenovirus is chosen as the primary virus that causes common cold?

Question two: why do influenza viruses HA and NA change?

What happens thereafter will be disclosed in Chapter 7.

Where are our unknown enemies?

Chapter 7

Variation

Flu viruses can also be classified as human influenza viruses and avian influenza viruses based on different host cells they infect. Antigens on the viral surface are "keys," while the receptors of host cells are "locks." Characteristics of "lock" and "key," namely, host species to be infected by viruses, are determined by spatial structures and physiochemical properties in different proteins.

1. Avian Flu

Sun Wukong, one of the protagonists in *Journey to the West*, which is one of the Four Great Classical Novels in China, is a stone monkey born of the essence of heaven and earth. He declared himself to be the Handsome Monkey King in the Cave of Water Curtains on the Mountains of Flowers and Fruits. He robbed the Magic Sea-Fixing Pin in the East Sea Dragon Palace, wrecking havoc in the sea, which disturbed the Heaven Palace. The Jade Emperor wanted to call upon the 100,000-strong heavenly army to set up a net in heaven and earth to capture him. However, the White Venus advised the Emperor to tame him with a position in the Heaven Palace in order to maintain peace in heaven and avoid war and disaster on earth. Thus, the stone monkey was conferred the name "Bima Wen."

Bima Wen shares a similar pronunciation with "avoiding the horses' plague" in Chinese. It is believed that a monkey put in a stable could effectively prevent horses from catching an illness. Thus, Sun Wukong was conferred the title "Bima Wen." Presumably that is why the "Great Sage Equal to Heaven" (a title boasted by Sun Wukong himself) later wrecked havoc in the Heaven Palace, which led to his punishment of being crushed under Five Elements Mountain for 500 years. Eventually, he was granted the great Fighting Buddha for his service and strength.

Equine plague, swine plague, fowl plague... all these are general terms to denote unknown animal diseases.

Edoardo Perroncito first described the highly pathogenic avian influenza in his publication in 1878. The poultry raised in Turin, Italy, had mild clinical symptoms at first, soon followed by highly pathogenic symptoms leading to the death of all poultry in this region. It was regarded as a devastating poultry disease. In 1901, Centanni and Savonuzzi confirmed that the disease was caused by a virus. However, it was not until 1955 that it was identified as an influenza virus.

In 1925, Beaudette still named this disease as fowl plague, which was renamed as Highly Pathogenic Avian Influenza (HPAI) in the First International Conference on Avian Influenza in 1981.

Avian Influenza (AI), an infection or disease syndrome caused by the Avian Influenza Virus (AIV), can lead to malignant infections and rapid deaths in poultry such as chickens, turkeys, etc. The AIV can result in severe infectious diseases in poultry, the mortality rate of which is 100%.

- In 1894, a severe, highly pathogenic avian influenza outbreak in Northern Italy spread to European countries such as Austria, Germany, France, Denmark, Czechoslovakia, and Poland, and continued for more than 40 years in Italy.
- In 1901, the highly pathogenic avian influenza was widespread throughout Germany during a poultry fair held in Braunschweig, Germany.
- In 1922, the highly pathogenic avian influenza epidemic also occurred in the UK and broke out in 1929.
- In 1924, the highly pathogenic avian influenza cases were reported in New York, Philadelphia, New Jersey, and other cities in the United States. In 1925, the epidemic spread to Virginia, Illinois, Michigan, and other states. In 1929, it attacked New Jersey once more.

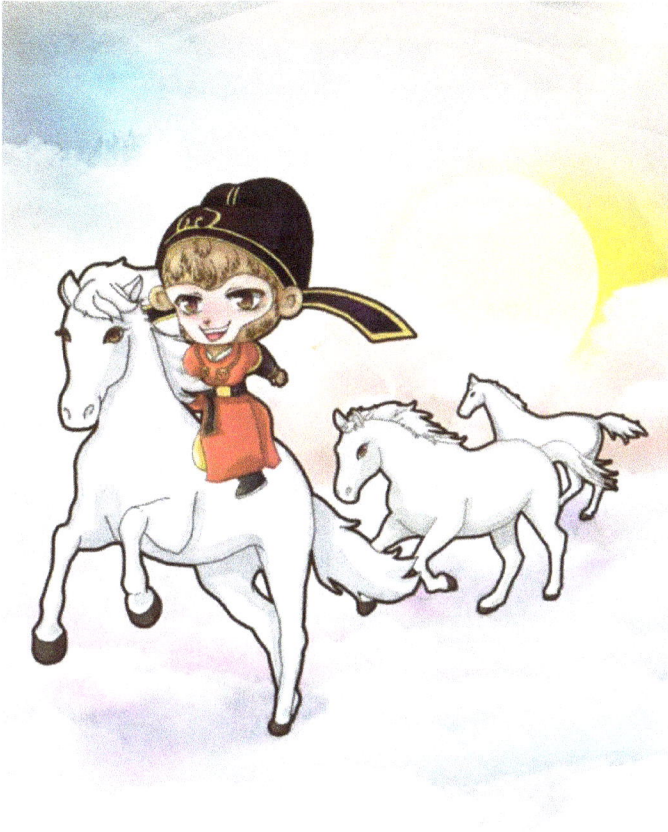

弼马温：趋避马瘟之意

Bima Wen: Avoiding Horses' Plague

- In 1961, thousands of seagulls in South Africa died of avian influenza virus.
- In 1983, the avian influenza virus outbreak in Ireland resulted in the culling of 30,000 chickens and 270,000 ducks; 17 million poultry were culled in the avian influenza epidemic in the United States in the same year.
- In 1995, the avian influenza virus outbreak in Mexico infected poultry in eleven states there; meanwhile, 3.2 million poultry were culled in the highly pathogenic avian influenza in Pakistan.

- In 1999, the highly pathogenic avian influenza occurred in Italy once more, which lasted until the following year, leading to deaths and culling of 13 million poultry.
- In 2003, the highly pathogenic avian influenza outbreak in Netherlands spread to Belgium and Germany, leading to the deaths and culling of 30 million poultry.
- In 2005, the avian influenza caused deaths of more than 6,000 wild migratory birds in Qinghai Lake in central China, including zebra geese, gulls, hemp ducks, and cormorants, which was the first global, large-scale deaths of migratory birds caused by avian influenza.

There are more than 30 pathogenic avian influenza recorded worldwide, among which, highly pathogenic avian influenza H5N1 has caused severe avian influenza epidemics in migratory birds in 63 countries in Asia, Europe, and Africa since 1996, including the one occurred in Qinghai Lake in central China in 2005, which infected 250 million poultry there. The spread of the highly pathogenic avian influenza not only brings great loss for poultry farmers but also requires the government to spend huge sums on infected poultry culling and public health protection.

The year of 2013 was a puzzling year humans and frightening one for birds.

The emergence of human infection with a new influenza virus H7N9 was reported in China. The first case of human infected H7N9 avian influenza was reported in Shanghai on February 19, 2013. By the end of April 2013, the number of infections has increased significantly, with a total of 125 confirmed cases mainly Jiangsu and Zhejiang provinces and Shanghai in eastern China. The second wave occurred in the autumn of 2013. There were 440 confirmed cases with 122 fatalities as of May 6, 2014. Since then, the virus has spread across the country, leading to more than 1,500 human infections and deaths.

Human H7N9 infection is a new, contagious, acute respiratory disease resulting from contact with infected poultry. Following an incubation period of seven days, human H7N9 infections present with such symptoms as acute fever and cough, which will quickly result in acute respiratory distress syndrome, severe pneumonia, and even death in severe cases.

Based on the analysis of clinical samples from patients, together with their clinical symptoms, laboratory pathological results, and epidemiological data, it is found that the pathogenic agent of the human influenza outbreak is a new H7N9 influenza A virus, a Low Pathogenic Avian Influenza Virus (LPAIV), with H7 hemagglutinin and N9 neuraminidase.

However, with the gene mutation of H7, LPAIV mutated into a Highly Pathogenic Avian Influenza Virus (HPAIV) since the summer of 2016, which infected humans in 2017. Particularly, the high or low pathogenicity only reflected by the virulence to chickens. Both LPAIV and HPAIV can cause diseases in humans.

H7N9 influenza is an alert sign for a new subtype of influenza virus spreading to threaten public health. In addition, virus variation may lead to a new influenza outbreak or a worldwide pandemic of infectious disease.

Avian influenza virus or human influenza virus, that is a question.

Why can H7N9 virus be transmitted from infected poultry to humans? Scientists have addressed the puzzling problem of virus mutation by exploring "tiny clues" of the mystery. The answer is that the emerging H7N9 influenza virus was produced with the genetic reassortment and variation of avian flu virus, and evolving "keys" to open the "locks" of human host cells.

2. Interspecies Transmission

The most confusing life has a starting point even if its origin may not be found. For example, we know at least that Sun Wukong, wreaking havoc in the Heaven Palace, jumped out of the stone into the East China Sea. As for H7N9 virus, at least the origins of H7 and N9 can be explored even if the origin of the virus is not traced back.

The whole genome of H7N9 virus contains its genetic information. It is found that its HA gene is highly similar to A/duck/12/2011 (H7) isolated from ducks in the Yangtze River Delta; its NA gene is highly homologous to A/wild bird/ Korea/ A14/2011 (N9), an emerging influenza virus.

How does influenza virus reassortment occur and realize interspecies transmission from duck and chicken hosts to humans?

Pigs have long been regarded as "mixers" for virus reassortment since human and avian viruses can coexist in pigs. With the progress of the cell life cycle, the reassortment and evolution of the genome fragments of viruses may produce new human influenza viruses. It is found in studies of origins of the H7N9 virus that viruses may directly reassort in infected chickens and evolve into new influenza viruses which can infect humans.

Thus, what happens to proteins of the influenza virus as it crosses species?

H7N9 virus, with typical characteristics and structure of influenza A virus, is a subtype of influenza A virus. When entering the host, the influenza virus first attaches to the cell and mediates its entry via binding hemagglutinin to cell receptor proteins. This "invasion" process determines the "key" and "lock" that influenza virus uses to identify cells among different species.

The main cell receptor of avian influenza HA protein is Gal-α2,3-sialyltransferase, while human influenza HA protein prefers Gal-α2,6-sialyltransferase. Thus, the "key" opens the particular "lock." The virus usually invades the upper respiratory tract, followed by the lower respiratory tract and even the lungs.

Receptors of the human upper respiratory tract are mainly Gal-α2,6-sialyltransferase, while receptors of the lower respiratory tract contain Gal-α2,3-sialyltransferase, similar to those in the poultry respiratory tract. Generally, it is not easy for the avian influenza virus to enter deep into the human lower respiratory tract. Even if it does arrive there, it will be trapped by tissue mucus, like falling into a "the cave of silken web," failing to escape to spread.

The novel genetic reassortant H7N9 virus, with characteristics of "dual receptor binding," enhances the binding of hemagglutinin to Gal-α2,6-sialyltransferase. Thus, it obtains the function of infecting cells in human upper respiratory tract. With the preference to binding to cell receptors in avian respiratory tract, the H7N9 virus has limited ability to transmit from person to person.

Influenza virus with different subtypes features high mutation rate and frequent gene reassortment. Even without "dozens of variations," there are 18 hemagglutinin and 11 neuraminidase subtypes in the known influenza A virus, which means there are 198 different ways to pair these two proteins and form different subtypes (or 16 HA to be paired with

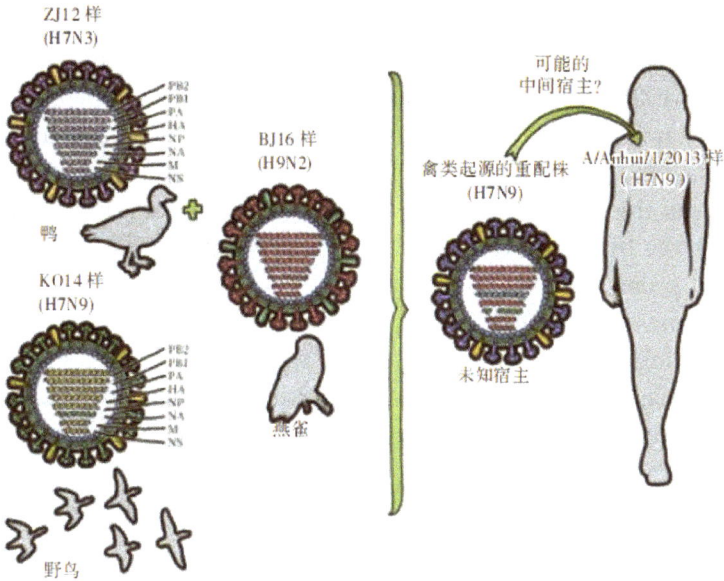

ZJ12 样
(H7N3)

BJ16 样
(H9N2)

可能的
中间宿主?

禽类起源的重配株
(H7N9)

A/Anhui/1/2013 样
(H7N9)

鸭

K014 样
(H7N9)

焦雀

未知宿主

野鸟

H7N9 流感病毒的流行、演化与跨种传播

Prevalence, Evolution, and Interspecies Transmission of H7N9 Influenza Virus

ZJ12-like (H7N3)

Ducks

K014-like (H7N9)

Wild birds

BJ16-like (H9N2)

Bramblings

Reassortant avian-origin (H7N9)

Unknown host

Possible intermediate hosts

A/Anhui/1/2013 (H7N9)-like

9 NA to form 144 subtypes when two bat viruses are excluded). It is already dazzling even if type B, C, and D have not been paired.

Why do the genes of influenza virus change so frequently? Reviewing the nature of viruses, it is known that adenovirus is a DNA virus, while influenza virus is an RNA virus. According to the Central Dogma, DNA encodes RNA, and RNA encodes protein.

The influenza virus is a negative-sense, single-stranded RNA virus [(-) (ssRNA)] that cannot be directly used as mRNA after entering the cell but uses (-)ssRNA as a template to transcribe the RNA complementary to it through transcriptase and then uses the complementary RNA as mRNA to translate the protein determined by the genetic code.

To put it simply: the double helix structure of DNA makes it more stable; by contrast, the single-stranded structure of RNA is more mutation-prone than that of DNA.

Influenza virus mutation mainly refers to antigenic variation. For example, influenza A virus' major surface antigen hemagglutinin and neuraminidase consist of amino acids with possible genetic code changes by both antigenic shift and antigenic drift.

Antigenic Shift

Antigenic shift is a qualitative process with large-scale mutations on the surface antigens of one or two virus strains to form a new subtype different from antigens of original strains. Antigenic shift may lead to changes in both HA antigen and NA antigen, or mutations in one of these two antigens and small or no changes for the other.

An influenza pandemic occurs since people lack the immunity to the mutated strain. Influenza A virus is the most frequently mutated type, with a large-scale antigenic mutation every dozen years to produce a new strain, such as the mutated virus subtypes H1N1, H2N2, and H3N2 in four influenza pandemics in human history.

Antigenic Drift

Antigenic drift is a quantitative process with small-scale or continuous variations, namely intra-subtype mutation. Among three influenza viruses infecting humans, influenza A virus has high mutation rates, followed by influenza B virus, while influenza C virus is relatively stable antigenically.

These variations are generally caused by genetic point mutations of the virus and selection of human immunity. Influenza virus only causes disease in a small cluster of humans. Mutations of influenza B virus can produce new strains. The immune response to original strains remains effective to new ones due to the cross immunity between them.

DNA is the essential hereditary material of humans, while most viruses have RNA as their genetic material. The reason perhaps lies in the fact that DNA ensures the stability of genetic information, while RNA can effectively change genetic information.

It seems that they are all evolutionary choices from the perspective of nature.

In addition to H7N9 virus, more than 60% of human diseases caused by viral infections originate from animals, such as SARS coronavirus and MERS coronavirus carried by bats, and Flavivirus and Zika virus carried by mosquitoes, all of which are likely to be transmitted to infect humans via vectors. It is our responsibility to maintain lucid waters and lush mountains for keeping healthy in a harmonious ecology.

3. Borders of Nature

From an evolutionary perspective, humans came much later than viruses. For viruses, humans are nothing more than one more choice in their host list, while for humans, viruses are just one more known entity in their lives.

Did viruses attack humans or humans invade their territory?

Ebola

In 1976, the headmaster of a local school at Yambuku town, Zaire (now Democratic Republic of Congo, DRC), died of fever in the hospital. Soon, several dozen patients developed a similar febrile hemorrhagic syndrome, which spread to 55 villages along the Ebola River soon, resulting in 280 deaths and an 88% mortality rate.

It was found in the WHO investigation that the cause of this disaster was an unprecedented pathogen — Ebola Virus (EBOV). The Ebola epidemic outbreak occurred in the neighboring Sudan and Ethiopia. Featuring abrupt onset and high fatality rate, the Ebola viral disease can be quickly

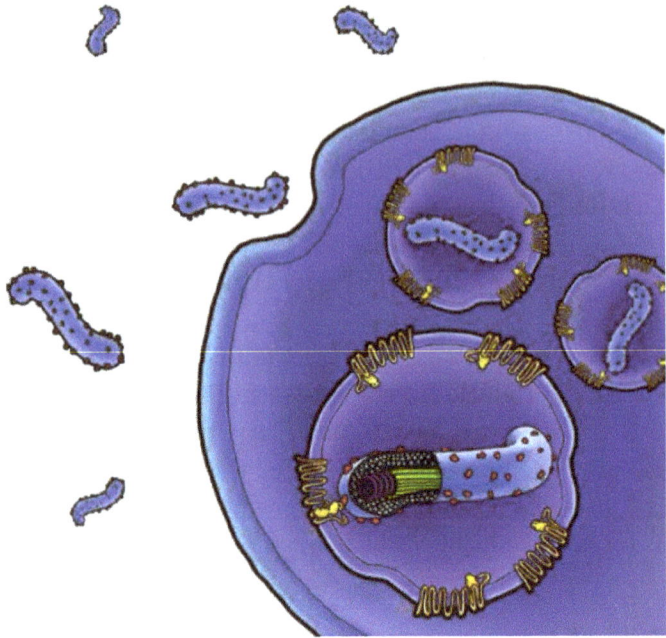

埃博拉病毒入侵细胞模式图

Ebola Virus Invading Host Cell

transmitted to humans, leading to acute bleeding and death in a short period of time. Many infected people died within three days after onset of illness. Within three months, a total of 602 people were infected and 431 died, resulting in a 72% mortality rate.

Ebola epidemic outbreaks occurred nearly simultaneously in Zaire and Sudan. The *Ebolavirus* genus consists of five distinct species based on outbreak locations, namely, *Zaire ebolavirus*, *Sudan ebolavirus*, *Reston ebolavirus*, *Tai Forest ebolavirus*, and *Bundibugyo ebolavirus*. *Reston ebolavirus* is the only ebolavirus that infects non-human primates via air. The other four ebolaviruses can infect humans, among which, *Zaire ebolavirus* is the most pathogenic, with case fatality rates as high as 90%.

From 1976 to 2013, 1,716 confirmed cases of ebolavirus diseases were reported by WHO. The Ebola outbreak in West Africa in March 2014 was the largest and most complex Ebola epidemic since its discovery.

There were more cases and deaths in this outbreak than all others combined. It was estimated that 14,000 people died worldwide due to the Ebola epidemics by March 10, 2015. A large number of cases remained unrecorded due to relatively underdeveloped health systems in the epidemic-affected areas.

Traces of Ebola virus were found by scientists in chimpanzees, monkeys, and other primates, as well as bats. Ebola viruses are generally transmitted from animal to animal, from animal to person, or from person to person via direct contact. Ebola hemorrhagic fever, an endemic infectious disease, rarely spreads to other areas outside Africa. However, the threat posed by Ebola virus will grow to be more pressing with the progress of globalization.

"SARS" and "Novel SARS"

In 2002, an atypical pneumonia (SARS) broke out in south China. In the following year, the Severe Acute Respiratory Syndrome, or SARS, was also detected in Guangdong province and Beijing. Then it spread soon to Australia, Canada, the US, and other corners of the world at an alarming speed.

The sudden global outbreak of this new disease, which killed many patients, including medical personnel, threw countless people into great panic.

On April 16, 2003, WHO officially announced that a new pathogen, the Severe Acute Respiratory Syndrome Coronavirus (also known as SARS coronavirus) is the cause of SARS. By August 7, 2003, there were 8,422 confirmed SARS cases and 919 deaths in 32 countries and regions across the world; China confirmed 5,327 cases and 349 deaths.

Bats were found to be the natural hosts of SARS-like coronavirus, the whole genome of which could be found in the viral genome database of bats. Viruses could be recombined to produce the direct ancestor of SARS coronavirus, making it possible to spread across species to humans.

In 2012, the first case of Middle East Respiratory Syndrome (MERS) was reported in Saudi Arabia. It was an infectious respiratory disease caused by the novel Middle East Respiratory Syndrome Coronavirus (MERS-CoV).

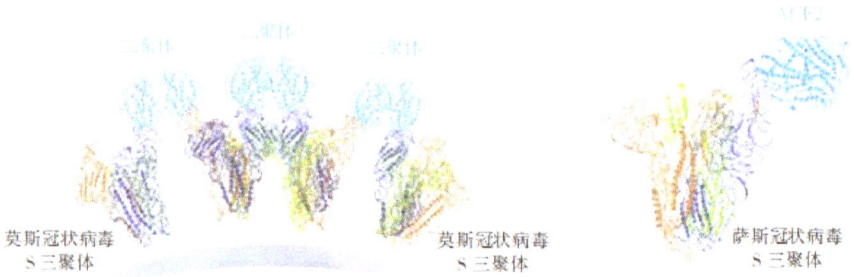

莫斯冠状病毒与萨斯冠状病毒虽同属冠状病毒，结合宿主细胞受体却不尽相同：CD26、ACE2

MERS-CoV S trimer

Dimer

Dimer

Dimer

MERS-CoV S trimer

SARS-CoV S trimer

Both MERS-CoV and SARS-CoV are coronaviruses, whereas they have different host cell binding receptors: CD26 and ACE2.

In 2015, MERS suddenly broke out in South Korea and spread rapidly, leading to the cancellation of public events, closure of over 2,400 schools, and quarantine of around 16,700 people. The MERS epidemic infected 186 people, leading to 36 deaths. Since the outbreak of the MERS epidemic, an infected patient from South Korea who entered China was confirmed in time and admitted to a hospital for emergency treatment. He was admitted to the ICU negative pressure room for treatment in isolation. The MERS entry alert was eventually lifted with emergency treatment for the infected and measures adopted such as disease surveillance and epidemic screening, disinfection and quarantine, and early warning for the public.

In 2018, a Korean returning from the Middle East was infected with MERS. Fortunately, that was the single imported case which did not spread to more humans.

In the 1960s, coronavirus was isolated and found to infect the respiratory system of humans, dogs, chickens, and other organisms. MERS-CoV, the sixth human coronavirus discovered, which shared similar genetic information with SARS-CoV, was called "novel SARS."

Camels have been regarded as the main source of food and leather by people in the Middle East for over a thousand years. More importantly, they were bestowed with the title "Ship of the Desert" for providing transportation and serving as pack animals for transporting goods. It is found that bats, which are natural hosts of MERS-CoV, transmit the virus to humans via dromedary camels as intermediate hosts.

Zika

In 1947, Zika Virus (ZIKV) was first identified in Uganda, where scientists conducted routine surveillance for yellow fever of monkeys. Suddenly, a monkey was noticed to develop fever. It was from this monkey that scientists isolated the virus and named it "Zika," meaning "grass" in Ugandan language.

The Zika virus epidemic broke out in Chile, Brazil, and other countries in 2015 and rapidly spread to the Americas, with an unprecedented increase in the number of infections. More than 4,000 cases of babies born with microcephaly were reported within half a year, which attracted the global attention.

On February 1, 2016, WHO held an emergency meeting to declare that "microcephaly" was caused by Zika virus outbreak and its transmission became a global public health emergency. Around 20% of people infected with Zika virus have mild symptoms, such as fever, rash, joint pain, and conjunctivitis, which lasts less than a week. However, Zika virus infection during pregnancy can cause infants to be born with microcephaly and even lead to death. It has been confirmed that Zika virus can directly cause microcephaly in infants.

Zika virus, an insect-borne virus transmitted by mosquitoes, mainly spreads among wild primates and mosquitoes living in trees, such as Aedes mosquitoes in Africa. It is relatively insidious, with sporadic infection cases in the equatorial regions in Asia, Africa, the Americas, and the Pacific. A total of 69 countries and territories have reported mosquito-borne Zika virus in the latest outbreak. In 2018, evidence for person-to-person transmission of Zika virus has been found by 11 countries including the US, France, Germany, and New Zealand.

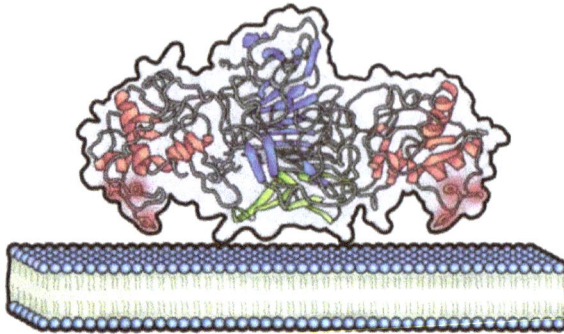

寨卡病毒 NS1 膜结合示意图

Zika Virus NS1 Contributes to Membrane Association

Another three Flaviviridae viruses can also be transmitted by Aedes mosquitoes, including Dengue virus, Chikungunya virus, and Flaviviruses, which cause epidemics in tropical and subtropical areas. Yellow fever virus, the first human virus discovered, is still listed as one of the quarantinable infectious diseases by WHO since it is a highly contagious virus with a high mortality rate.

Chimpanzees, monkeys, bats, camels, and mosquitoes are all integral components of living systems in nature. It is impossible for humans to live alone on earth. Viruses mutate in order to better adapt to their hosts, cells develop acquired immunity with the purpose of better protecting the body, and living organisms evolve so as to better engage in the environment.

In the process of our transformation of nature, the deeper we look into nature, the more we recognize that the unknown world is larger and more complex than we thought. As an old saying in *the Book of Changes* goes, "What is above form is called Dao, and what is under form is called 'an object,'" which means above or beyond the form is the abstract natural law, whereas within the form is concrete. In the micro war without smoke between humans and viruses, new "objects" are needed to be developed and upgraded constantly to resist virus attack and protect our health; while in the sharing of peaceful coexistence between living and non-living things, biodiversity "Dao" should be followed to maintain the balance of nature and keep the ecological harmony.

What can we do to fight enemies?

Chapter 8

Cause and Effect

"To nip something in the bud" is the best measure of protection. Early detection of diseases buys time for the cells fighting to restore health. More importantly, undoubtedly the most effective measurement of disease prevention and control is the timely detection of the infection source and cutting off the transmission route at the early stage during a serious epidemic. As a Chinese saying goes, "He who has a thorough knowledge of the enemy and himself" will be "as stable as Mount Tai."

1. Origin

The incubation period of H7N9 influenza virus generally ranges from one to seven days, with an average of two to four days.

Most people infected with the H7N9 virus show symptoms such as fever (39–40°C), headache, muscle pain, general malaise, chills, systemic muscle and joint pain, tiredness, loss of appetite, sore throat, cough, nasal congestion, runny nose, retrosternal pain, flushed cheeks, and conjunctival congestion. Children infected with influenza B virus generally have symptoms such as vomiting, abdominal pain, and diarrhea.

Infected patients without complications generally experience the self-limiting disease recovery course. The body temperature usually returns to normal and systemic symptoms are relieved in three or four days after the onset of illness. However, it takes one to two weeks to recover from cough and regain physical strength.

It is good to recover from influenza complications through medical treatment; it is better for those infected without complications to recover on their own, but it is best to track virus traces during the incubation period and monitor individual health in advance so as to improve the chances of conquering the disease.

Imagine boldly: how about discovering sources of infection before the viruses attack us. This is the concept behind "tracing viruses' origins."

In the superhero world, with an ever-overcast night sky, a dark knight wears a high-tech black battle armor and helmet as well as his iconic black batwing cape and drives a sports vehicle at full speed whizzing through the night in a metropolitan city. He instills fear in his enemies, making them tremble at the sight of the shadows of bats in the night sky. The knight is "the Batman."

A group of scientists from cities, wearing white biosecurity suits as well as safety glasses and gloves, take biological sampling tools to explore the secrets of bats in jungles and caves, in the hope of tracing the origin of SARS, which once brought great fear to humans.

In 2002, Severe Acute Respiratory Syndrome Coronavirus (SARS Coronavirus) suddenly attacked humans. It broke out in China, swept the whole world in 2003, and abruptly disappeared without a trace. Those lucky enough to escape this "plague" always ask the question: where did the virus come from, and where is it going?

Like the interspecies transmission of avian influenza, people's prime suspect is wild animal, the most relevant to the SARS pandemic. Soon, civet became the prime suspect, since the earliest identified cases of SARS in Guangdong province were mainly wildlife cooks and staff working in the wildlife market, who were always in direct contact with civets.

Soon, it was found in the investigation that SARS Coronavirus, which was detected in civets in the wildlife market, had highly consistent (99.8%) whole genome sequence with those spreading to people. The evidence is enough to prove that civets were "accomplices" in transmitting the virus to humans.

We only call civets "accomplices," since it is found in animal studies that SARS Coronavirus not only causes diseases in humans but also in civets, which means civets are also "victims" of the virus; moreover, there is no evidence of naturally infected civets in epidemiological studies on either wild or domestic civets. Does it mean that civets are merely "transitional" intermediate hosts?

As a "marginal life" completely parasitizing the host, the virus itself will face the end of life if it causes diseases or even deaths in all its hosts. Thus, there are always some natural hosts for virus to co-exist in nature, achieving a state of equilibrium between species, like the gut flora in our body. These hosts may be the true "origin" of the virus.

Bats flying at night are pterodactyls found all over the world.

In the long-time evolutionary process, bats have developed a special immune system, which protects them from diseases even though they carry various viruses. As a result, bats have become natural "reservoirs" for many viruses such as Ebola virus, Hendra virus, rabies virus, etc. Scientists previously have found that bats transmitted viruses they carried to humans via pigs, horses, dogs, and other animals. Are bats natural hosts of SARS Coronavirus?

How can we know whether it is true or not if we do not catch a few bats?

In 2005, scientists found that bats are natural hosts of SARS-like Coronaviruses, whose family member SARS Coronavirus led to SARS outbreak in humans. Researchers spent over two years studying bats in Guangdong province, Guangxi Zhuang Autonomous Region, Hubei province, and Tianjin municipality, China. They detected antibodies to SARS Coronavirus in bats and proved bats to be the origin of SARS virus from the genetic level since genes in one of the bat coronavirus strains was highly consistent (92%) with those in viruses infecting humans and civets. More than 400 biological bat samples contributed to this discovery.

In 2013, researchers isolated the first live SARS-like coronavirus strain from bat samples, which resembled the SARS strain more closely than those previously identified in bats. The membrane S (spike) protein on the surface of the SARS virus particle, which is the receptor-binding protein of the host cell, is "Mr. Key" to help the virus enter the host cell. The findings were achieved by identifying the same receptors between the newly discovered virus and SARS viruses as well as its infections of human cells, which confirmed the "living origin" of SARS virus at the cellular level. It took another eight years of unremitting efforts to track traces of the virus in bats in spring and autumn.

In 2017, research teams found all the genetic information of SARS virus in 15 strains of SARS-like coronavirus collected in bats, though none of strains were completely identical to the SARS virus. Through the calculation and analysis of viral genetic recombination information data, frequent recombination was detected in multiple sites of genomes and over 97% similarity was determined between them. They suggested the possible recombination of origins of SARS Coronavirus: SARS virus parasitizing bats jumped to civets and then was passed on to humans; or SARS-like coronavirus parasitizing bats infected civets and recombined into SARS virus within civets, and then was transmitted to humans. It took five years to accomplish the full evidence chain of "information source."

Fifteen years of scientific research contributed to establishing the source of SARS coronavirus, similar to burning a torch of knowledge in a dark cave to illuminate the road to progress for humans to explore the unknown nature and "catch" hiding "criminals."

Human growth is like the metamorphosis of Batman, who fell into a deep well in a castle at an early age, where countless bats in the dark brought him great fear. Escaping would only bring more fear. Only by overcoming the fear in our mind could we turn into the true "Batman."

Anyone can conquer his fear but cannot eliminate it; similarly, humans may defeat viruses but cannot wipe out them. A person who is detected at the early stage of viral infection can improve clinical treatment efficiency; a region where viruses are discovered at the early stage can provide a better public health environment; a country where viruses are discovered at the early stage can take measures to prevent and control diseases; and a world where viruses are discovered at the early stage can ensure the health of all humans.

There is a common misconception that if someone catches a cold, he should first take a handful of antibiotics. However, antibiotics are designed for bacterial infections, while viral infections should be treated with anti-viral drugs. "Diagnosis" must be the prerequisite for "treatment," no matter how different the methods of Eastern and Western medicine are. Only by identifying the "cause" of the disease can we cure it.

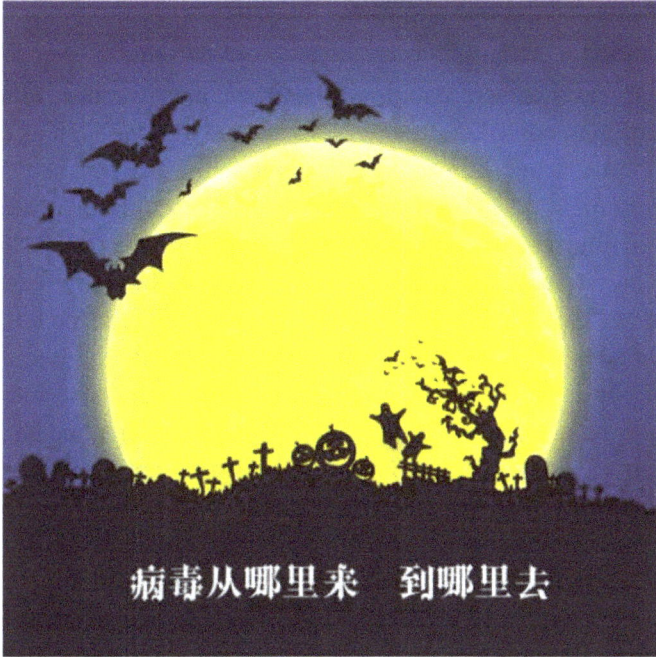

萨斯病毒溯源：蝙蝠

Where is Virus From? Where is Virus Headed To?
Bats are the Origin of SARS-CoV

2. "Crime Scene"

H7N9 virus diagnosis is usually made based on the clinical and laboratory diagnosis. The former includes clinical epidemiological history inquiry, clinical symptom observations, and imaging examination; the latter generally refers to blood analysis and rapid diagnostic testing. Confirmatory tests depend on serologic tests, viral nucleic acid tests, viral isolation and culture, etc.

Clinical Diagnosis

Pneumonia is the most common influenza complication. Most people infected with flu show mild symptoms and will not develop pneumonia.

Their influenza symptoms will further aggravate in two to four days after the onset of illness or in late stages of recovery. The following symptoms may appear: fever, severe cough, purulent sputum, dyspnea, moist rales, and signs of lung consolidation; nervous system injuries such as encephalitis, meningitis, acute necrotizing encephalopathy, myelitis, and Guillain–Barré syndrome; and occasional heart injuries such as myocarditis and pericarditis. Elevated levels of creatine kinase and abnormal electrocardiogram can be observed in the clinical diagnosis. In severe cases, heart failure may occur, leading to significantly increased risk for hospitalization and deaths associated with myocardial infarction, ischemic heart disease; myositis and rhabdomyolysis are mainly manifested by myalgia, myasthenia, renal failure, elevated levels of serum creatine kinase and myoglobin, and acute kidney injury, etc., whereas septic shock is characterized by fever, shock, and multiple organ dysfunctions.

Imaging examinations of patient with complicated pneumonia showed patchy, ground-glass shadow, and exudative lesions in multiple lobes; in the advanced stage, both lungs are shown with diffuse exudative lesions or consolidation, and pleural effusion is seen in a few cases. The patchy shadows in lungs appear earlier in infected children, with multiple and scattered distribution, which are prone to over-aeration. Their imaging manifestations change rapidly, such as the progressive expansion and fusion of lesions, leading to pneumothorax and mediastinal emphysema.

Laboratory Diagnosis

In the regular examination of peripheral blood of patients, the total white blood cell count is generally not high or even lower than the normal value, and the number of lymphocytes is significantly lower than normal range in severe cases; in blood biochemical examination, hypokalemia may occur in some cases, and a few cases may show elevated levels of creatine kinase, aspartate aminotransferase, alanine aminotransferase, lactate dehydrogenase, creatinine, etc.

Colloidal gold and immunofluorescence methods can be used for rapid antigen testing. The interpretation of the rapid antigen test should integrate the patient's epidemiological history and clinical symptoms since the sensitivity of the rapid antigen test is lower than that of the nucleic acid test.

The diagnosis can be confirmed based on the above clinical flu manifestations in clinical and laboratory tests, together with the following positive test results.

- Serological test: to detect the level of IgM and IgG antibody specific to influenza virus. There is retrospective diagnostic significance when the level of IgG antibody detected dynamically in the recovery period is four times or higher than that in the acute period.
- Viral nucleic acid detection: RT-PCR (real-time RT-PCR is preferred) is used to detect influenza virus nucleic acids in respiratory specimens (pharyngeal swabs, nasal swabs, nasopharyngeal or tracheal extracts, sputum). With the best specificity and sensitivity, viral nucleic acid detection can identify virus types and subtypes. With the popularization of genetic sequencing techniques, the sequencing of PRC products is also widely used.
- Virus isolation and culture: influenza virus is isolated from respiratory specimens. In the influenza season, it is suggested that viruses should also be isolated from those patients with negative results for the rapid antigen detection of influenza-like cases and immunofluorescence test.

To sum up, test results should involve "three elements": protein, nucleic acid, and live virus, which is particularly manifested by four times or higher levels of IgG antibody specific to influenza virus in the recovery period than that in the acute period in serological tests, positive results of virus nucleic acids in real-time RT-PCR or RT-PCR, and positive results of virus isolation and culture.

The Naming of Antibodies: Immunoglobulin

The Special Committees of WHO and International Union of Immunological Societies decided to name the globulin with antibody activity or chemical structure similar to antibody as immunoglobulin (Ig) in 1968 and 1972, respectively. Ig is the concept related to chemical structure, while antibody is the term associated with biological function. The chemical fundamental of all antibodies is Ig, while Ig does not have a direct role in the antibody activity.

A natural Ig molecule contains identical amino acid compositions in its two H chains and two L chains. Various Ig H chain constant regions contain different compositions and sequences of amino acids, leading to their disparate antigenicity, based on which, there are five Ig classes or isotypes:

IgM, IgD, IgG, IgA, IgE.

IgG is the main type of antibody found in blood and extracellular fluid, representing approximately 75%–80% of serum antibodies in humans. It is the main antibody produced by human immune response. Featuring strong affinity and wide distribution in the body, IgG, the "main force" to guard the body against infection, has an important immune effect: IgG can play an important role in the newborn's anti-infection immunity by crossing the human placenta.

IgM is the Ig with the highest molecular weight, also referred to as macroglobulin, accounting for 5%–10% of serum immunoglobulin in humans. Mainly found in blood, IgM has strong antigen-binding ability and cannot easily pass through the blood vessel walls. IgM, the body's "vanguard" of fighting infection, is the first antibody to appear in the humoral immune response. The presence of IgM in serum indicates recently acquired infection, which can be used for the early diagnosis of infection.

IgA can be divided into two types: serum type, mainly found in serum, represents 10%–15% of serum immunoglobulin in humans, whereas secretory IgA (SIgA) is mainly found in secretions from gastrointestinal and bronchial tracts, colostrum, saliva, and tears. As the primary antibody in exudates, SigA is involved in local mucosal immunity. It plays a vital role in local anti-infection by preventing pathogens from attaching to the cell surface by binding to the corresponding pathogenic microbes (bacteria, viruses, etc.).

IgD, which can be produced at any time of ontogenesis, is found in very small amounts in the serum of humans, merely representing 0.2% serum Ig in humans. IgE, with an extremely low concentration of about 5×10^{-5} mg/ml, is the Ig with the smallest amounts in normal human serum. As a pro-cell antibody, IgE can cause an allergic reaction by binding to high-affinity receptors on mast cells and basophils.

Therefore, the immune system will activate its response when the body is infected with the influenza virus. The detection of specific influenza virus IgM in early diagnosis can give us the message that "the virus came here just now"; as the major viral infection Ig is widely distributed, the detection of IgG can indicate that "the virus is still in the body." In particular, four times or even higher increase in IgG levels clearly indicate that the body is engaged in "fighting the virus."

Proteins, which serve as carriers of virus functions, are the main antigens produced by antibodies and stimulating antibodies. Specific

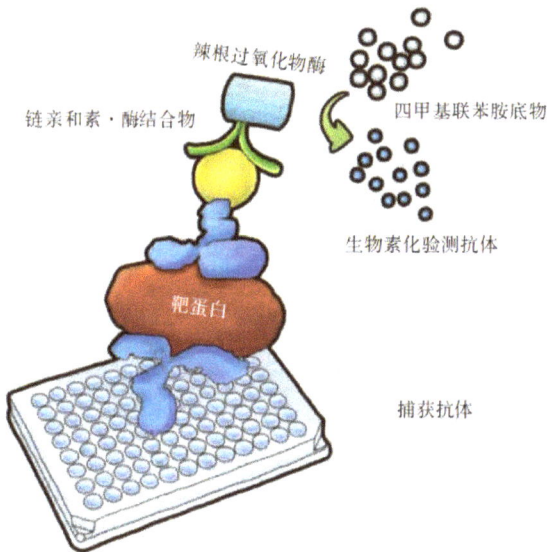

辣根过氧化物酶
链亲和素·酶结合物
四甲基联苯胺底物
生物素化验测抗体
靶蛋白
捕获抗体

酶联免疫吸附测定法（Enzyme Linked Immunosorbent Assay, ELISA）

Streptavidin. Enzyme combination

Horseradish peroxidase

Tetramethylbenzidine substrate

Biotin assay detecting antibodies

Antibodies capture

Target proteins

Enzyme-Linked Immunosorbent Assay (ELISA)

antigens induce their corresponding antibodies. The human body can be confirmed as infected with influenza virus when the flu "key" matches the "lock" of human Ig.

The Fingerprint of Nucleic Acids: Real-time RT-PCR and RT-PCR

Real-time RT-PCR, RT-PCR, and PCR refer to DNA synthesis polymerase chain reaction (PCR), reverse transcription polymerase chain reaction (RT-PCR), and real-time quantitative reverse transcription polymerase chain reaction (RQ-RT-PCR) in reverse order, respectively.

RT-PCR is an extension of PCR technology. In RT-PCR, the RNA molecule is reverse transcribed into a DNA molecule with complementary base pairing. Uracil (U) in the RNA molecule is converted into thymine (T) in the DNA molecule in this process. The complementary DNA is then used as a template for amplification via PCR. The important process of reverse transcription from RNA to DNA is achieved by an active protein enzyme called reverse transcriptase (RT).

In 1970, when studying cancer cells, Howard Temin and other scientists were puzzled about the flow of genetic information only from DNA to RNA. Howard Temin believed that circuits are likely to exist since some enzymes might have special functions. He found a special DNA polymerase in RNA viruses that are capable of causing cancer. Following base pairing, the enzyme uses RNA as a template to make a single-strand DNA complementary to it, which is called complementary DNA (cDNA).

This remarkable discovery, based on a particular type of RNA virus, retrovirus, upgrades the theoretical architecture of the Central Dogma. Retroviruses have a long incubation period and usually cause tumors in humans and animals, including AIDS triggered by HIV, leukemia virus, sarcoma virus, etc.

The nucleic acid of the retrovirus is composed of single-stranded RNA. The complementary negative-stranded DNA is synthesized by the reverse transcriptase using the viral RNA as a template, and double-stranded DNA is synthesized by the DNA polymerase. Then the viral DNA is integrated to the genomic DNA of the host cell and continuously reproduces itself to pass on to the daughter cells; DNA may also be transcribed into RNA, which continues to synthesize daughter virions. Only in the host cell division cycle can the DNA genome of retrovirus integrate

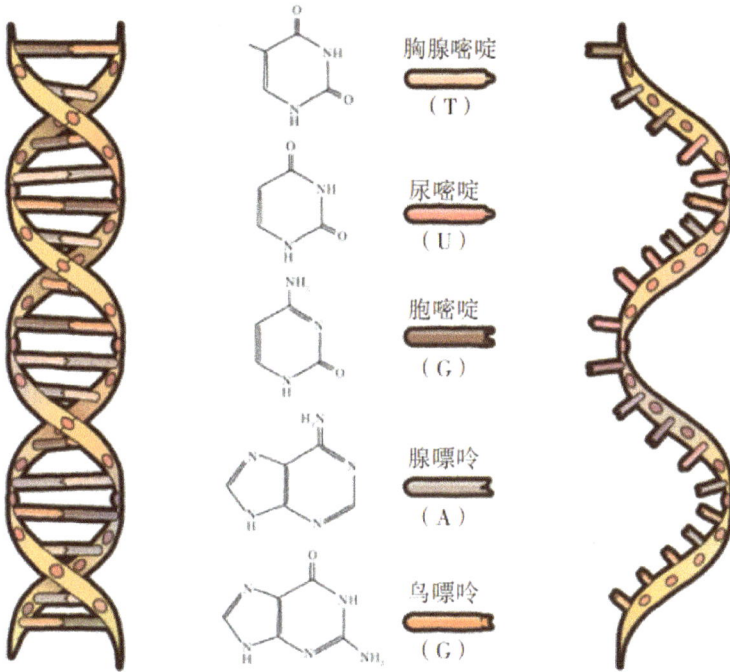

胸腺嘧啶
（T）

尿嘧啶
（U）

胞嘧啶
（G）

腺嘌呤
（A）

鸟嘌呤
（G）

DNA（左）和 RNA（右）的分子结构

Thymine (T)

Uracil (U)

Cytosine (C)

Adenine (A)

Guanine (G)

Molecular Structure of DNA (left) and RNA (right)

itself into the genetic material of the host cell and replicate itself in the dividing cell.

As RNA viruses, influenza viruses have RNA molecules as the genetic material. Therefore, it is necessary to reversely transcribe the genetic material, i.e., the viral RNA, to DNA and then amplify DNA molecule to the detection level so as to identify the "bio-fingerprint" of the viral nucleic acid. The reverse transcriptase is derived from the viral RNA.

Real-time RT-PCR, or real-time quantitative reverse transcription PCR, performs total or relative quantitative analysis of unknown templates via the standard curve. As a highly sensitive technology for RNA detection, real-time RT-PCR finds its wide application in the detection and diagnosis of diseases.

Based on RT-PCR technique with a few improvements, real-time RT-PCR develops fluorophore into the PCR reaction system to monitor the entire real-time PCR process by cumulative fluorescent signals. It uses the quantitative method to calculate and analyze the unknown template by studying the standard curve and mathematical model. It is due to the development of fluorescence signals and computational models in real-time RT-PCR that the subtle evidence of influenza virus RNA can be found in samples via data analysis even with small quantities of RNA.

The high-throughput screening (HTS) fluorescence analysis technique was developed based on real-time RT-PCR. Different markers of nucleic acid detection were designed in it according to genotype characteristics of disparate influenza viruses. Under relative conditions, HTS fluorescence analysis technique makes it possible to detect multiple samples at one time or carry out multiple detections for the same sample, which made PCR technique more specific, efficient, and accurate.

Nucleic acid serves as the carrier of virus information. The specific RNA sequence corresponds to the particular DNA sequence. Human infection with influenza virus will be confirmed when DNA sequence is amplified or captured by fluorescent signals in viral samples after the reverse transcription from viral RNA sequence.

The Living Evidence From a Crime Scene: Virus Culture and Isolation

Koch's Postulates, which are a set of common procedures used to determine an infectious disease, were initially mainly used for the discovery of bacteria and later applied to virus discovery, which, however, was more difficult to achieve.

As single-celled organisms, bacteria can replicate themselves and generate daughter cells through the use of nutrients in the environment, while viruses must live in hosts. Thus, the primary problem to solve is the host if we want to culture and isolate viruses.

As a diagnostic method, there are some limitations in virus isolation since limited strains of mammalian cell lines are available for virus culture. Appropriate cell lines are needed for virus culture in the laboratory, among which, MDCK cell lines are widely used in the amplification and purification of many viruses.

Derived by Madin and Darby from the kidney tissue of an adult female cocker spaniel, the MDCK cell line was established in 1958 and used as a model for studying epithelial growth through adhering to cell walls. It can be used in the culture of such viruses as reovirus, adenovirus, canine parvovirus, and influenza virus. Featuring high efficiency, rapid proliferation, and stable structure, it is universally acknowledged that the MDCK cell line is one of the three most suitable cell lines for producing influenza A and B vaccines.

Chicken embryo, just as its name implies, is the embryo of a chicken. Plato was challenged by Diogenes with a plucked chicken for his definition of man as "featherless bipeds"; Aristotle used chicken embryos to make contributions to the study of life development. Influenza viruses are suitable to be cultivated in chicken embryos, so are most avian viruses. Inoculated into the allantoic cavity of the chicken embryo of the right age, the virus can be propagated in the chicken embryo, producing live viruses, which can serve as a highly sensitive and efficient cell culture system for virus isolation.

As a basic life form, a particular virus has its host range. Human infection with influenza virus will be confirmed when the live influenza virus is isolated from cultured cell lines or chicken embryos.

The central principle remains the same. To obtain the direct evidence of the virus, it is necessary to start from the virus itself by "catching" its "original form."

Scientific solutions are necessary for the treatment of patients, so is for the prevention and control of diseases, "treatment" and "prevention" complement each other. Oseltamivir, a neuraminidase inhibitor, can treat influenza patients by preventing the release of influenza virions from host cells.

3. Measurement

There are three general types of influenza treatment: symptomatic treatment, antiviral treatment, and intensive care treatment.

Symptomatic treatment refers to providing physical cooling or antipyretics for treating fever; giving antitussive and expectorant drugs for treating severe cough and phlegm; offering nasal catheter, open face mask, and oxygen storage mask for oxygen therapy according to the degree of hypoxia; and appropriate use of antibiotics and other general therapy based on clinical symptoms for treating bacterial infections such as secondary bacterial pneumonia following influenza.

Intensive care treatment follows the principle of active treatment of primary disease, prevention and treatment of complications, and effective support for organ function. For example, if hypoxemia or respiratory failure occur, appropriate treatment measures should be adopted in time, such as oxygen therapy or mechanical ventilation; corresponding antishock treatment should be given for associated shocks; and related support treatment and other anti-infection measures should be undertaken at the occurrence of other visceral dysfunctions.

Antiviral treatment within 48 hours of onset can reduce complications of influenza, decrease the fatality rate of patients admitted to hospital, and shorten the duration of hospitalization. Patients with severe illness can still benefit from antiviral treatment more than 48 hours after illness onset, while high-risk groups for flu and patients with severe influenza should be given influenza antiviral treatment as early as possible (48 hours after illness onset) without waiting for virus test results. Antiviral treatment should also be given if symptoms are not alleviated or even worsen over 48 hours after illness onset. Besides, other patients can also receive antiviral treatment less than 48 hours after illness onset to shorten disease course and reduce complications.

Among influenza antiviral drugs, Tamiflu, which is familiar to us, is more famous for its simple name than its wide range of use. The full name of Tamiflu is Oseltamivir Capsule Phosphate, namely Oseltamivir.

These drugs are collectively known as neuraminidase inhibitors (NAIs), which can prevent the replication and release of daughter virions in human cells by selectively inhibiting neuraminidase activity on the viral surface of the respiratory tract.

Featuring antiviral efficiency, low drug resistance, and desirable drug tolerance, NAIs can effectively prevent cold and alleviate symptoms. It can obviously shorten the length of influenza if taken within 48 hours after the illness onset.

Oseltamivir, Zanamivir, Peramivir, Laninamivir are NAIs that are effective in fighting influenza A and B viruses. Amantadine and Rimantadine (M2 ion channel blockers) can only fight against influenza A virus. However, it is not recommended to use Amantadine and Rimantadine since it is shown in the current monitoring data that the influenza A virus is resistant to these drugs.

Do you have the same feeling for "vir," the suffix of the four drug names?

The term "intervention," most commonly used in medical treatment, particularly in psychology, refers to the process of exerting influences on psychological activities, individual characteristics, or psychological problems as planned step by step to secure a desired result. Application of this term to a community refers to the governance of health protection and disease control, and to a country refers to the law, the cornerstone of a state governance.

Law of the People's Republic of China on Prevention and Treatment of Infectious Diseases was adopted and revised by the Standing Committee of the Tenth National People's Congress, which took effect on December 1, 2004. The highly pathogenic avian influenza is explicitly included into infectious diseases under Class B. In addition, with respect to the highly pathogenic avian influenza of infectious diseases under Class B, measures for prevention and control of infectious diseases under Class A, as mentioned in the law, shall be taken.

Unsurprisingly, highly pathogenic avian influenza was included into the "highest levels of threat" list. How do we deal with the crisis? Let us see the stipulations of the law.

The "nets above and snares below" approach was established for disease prevention and control by institutions of disease prevention and control, medical agencies, and the society.

- Institutions of Disease Prevention and Control at all levels shall do the work of monitoring and forecasting infectious diseases, and of making epidemiological investigations and reporting on epidemic situations as well as the work of preventing and controlling other diseases.
- Medical agencies shall do the work of preventing and treating infectious diseases that is related to medical treatment and the work of preventing infectious diseases within their own responsibilities.

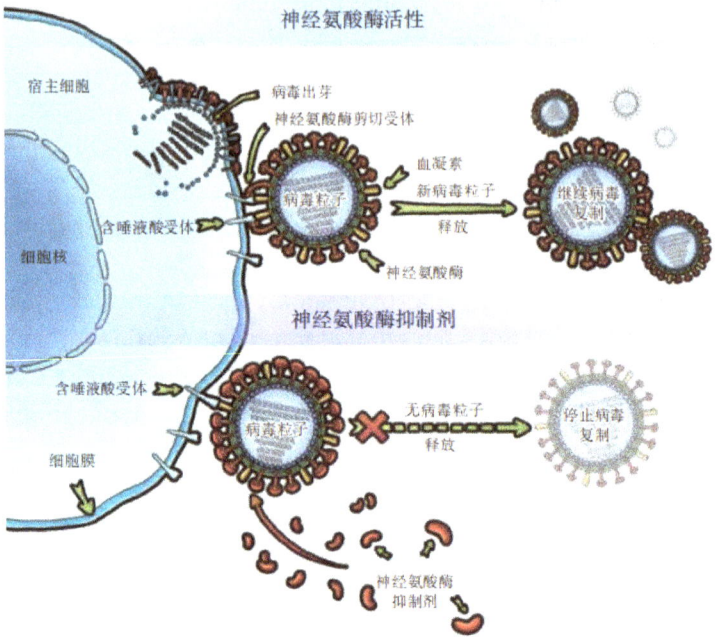

神经氨酸酶活性

宿主细胞　病毒出芽　神经氨酸酶剪切受体

血凝素　新病毒粒子　释放

病毒粒子　神经氨酸酶

继续病毒复制

含唾液酸受体

细胞核

神经氨酸酶抑制剂

含唾液酸受体　无病毒粒子　释放　停止病毒复制

病毒粒子

细胞膜

神经氨酸酶抑制剂

抗流感病毒药物·神经氨酸酶抑制剂

Nucleus	HA
Host cell	New virion
Receptor containing sialic acid	Release
Receptor containing sialic acid	NA
Cell membrane	No virion
NA activity	Release
Budding virus	NA inhibitors
NA cleaves receptor	Continued viral replication
Virion	Halted viral replication
NA inhibitors	Anti-influenza viral drugs: NA inhibitors
Virion	

- Units and individuals are encouraged to participate in the work of preventing and treating infectious diseases.

The "indirect hazards" that may cause disease transmission shall be cut off in an all-round way from such aspects as environment, transportation, and water resources.

- To improve environmental sanitation and eliminate hazards of rodents and vector organisms such as mosquitoes and flies.
- To eliminate hazards of rodents and schistosomiasis from farmlands, lake regions, rivers, livestock farms, and forest regions as well as hazards of other animals and vector organisms that transmit infectious diseases.
- To eliminate hazards of rodents and vector organisms such as mosquitoes and flies from means of transport and relevant places.
- To improve sanitary conditions of drinking water and take measures for the harmless disposal of sewage and waste.

Transmission regions of "land, sea, and air" should be controlled to minimum areas in terms of personnel, materials, animals, etc.

- Patients with infectious diseases, pathogen carriers, and suspected infectious victims shall, before they are cured or cleared of suspicion, be barred from jobs which laws or administrative regulations or the health administration department under the State Council prohibit them from doing due to the likelihood of causing the spread of infectious diseases.
- In the event of an outbreak of a Class A infectious disease, quarantine inspection of persons, goods and materials, and means of transport entering or leaving the epidemic area shall be conducted for the purpose of preventing the spread of the infectious disease.
- Quarantine measures for specific places where the infectious disease under Class A occurred and persons in particular areas in these places shall be formulated and approved. Living necessities shall be provided for persons in isolation. The termination of quarantine measures shall be determined and announced by authorities that originally made the decision.
- Measures should be taken to prevent, control, and administer zoonotic diseases related to infectious diseases common to human beings and animals.

The "hazard scope" of pathogens of infectious diseases shall be controlled and early warnings shall be issued by means of investigation, testing, monitoring, etc.

- In the event of the outbreak of an infectious disease, specialized technical institutions are admitted to conduct investigation, sample collection, technical analysis, and inspection in the epidemic site or area.
- Disease prevention and control institutions at different levels shall monitor the outbreak and prevalence of infectious diseases as well as factors affecting their outbreak and prevalence; and they shall monitor infectious diseases which have broken out abroad but have not yet spread at home or have newly began spreading at home.
- On the basis of the forecast of outbreak and epidemic trend of infectious diseases, the early warning of infectious diseases shall be issued in a timely manner and announcement shall be made depending on circumstances.
- A preliminary plan for prevention and control of infectious diseases shall be formulated and corresponding measures for prevention and control shall be adopted.

The "biosafety" of laboratories shall be ensured by medical agencies, disease prevention and control institutions, institutes, etc.

- Medical agencies shall strictly adhere to the control system and operation procedures to prevent iatrogenic and hospital infection of infectious diseases.
- Laboratories of disease prevention and control institutions and medical agencies as well as units engaged in experimentation of pathogenic microorganisms shall exercise strict supervision and control over pathogens samples of infectious diseases to strictly prevent the laboratory infection of pathogens of infectious diseases and spread of pathogenic microorganisms.
- The collection, preservation, carrying, transportation, and use of bacterial and viral strains of infectious diseases and samples of infectious diseases for testing shall be controlled in a classified manner, and a sound and rigorous control system shall be established.
- Where it is really necessary to collect, preserve, carry, transport, or use bacterial and viral strains of infectious diseases and samples of infectious diseases for testing that may cause the spread of the infectious diseases under Class A, the matter shall be subject to approval.

The disease prevention and control governance system will be fully established by following basic stipulations of the Law, including timely detection and early warning to cut off the risk of epidemic transmission, systematic detection and monitoring system and a preliminary plan for prevention and control, and sanitary disposal fully covering disease infection sources from different regions.

Without effective disease prevention and control, an infectious disease will continue to spread, which will create an unbearable burden on medical agencies. Without appropriate treatment, the infected patients will develop more serious disease and even die, which will turn disease prevention and control governance bodies into passive spectators and result in heavy casualties and trauma.

Influenza treatment requires "early detection, early diagnosis, early intervention, and early treatment." However, in fact, more can be done earlier than the aforementioned "four early."

What kind of weapons do we have to fight enemies?

Chapter 9

Bidding Game

Inactivated vaccines are the main vaccines used against influenza viruses in China at present. Featuring easy production and preservation, inactivated vaccines, as well as subunit vaccines, are also most commonly used worldwide. By reserving antigenic components of the influenza virus, a specific viral vaccine can be designed with a particular immune antigen.

1. Vaccine

Vaccines were "gifts" from cows in the past. What are the "functions" of vaccines at present?

The function of the vaccine is to trigger the body to produce an immune response to a pathogen's antigen. With immunogenicity and immunoactivity, it is a special antigen that can induce specific immune response in the body and combine specifically with antibodies for reaction.

- The antigen is any substance that induces an immune response. All immunogenic substances are antigenic.
- Substances that are antigenic but not immunogenic will not provoke an immune response in the body.

Live Attenuated Vaccines

People have been searching for the "gift" of nature for a long time since the invention of vaccinia vaccine. It was not until the discovery of micro-organisms and the proposal that germs lead to diseases when people fully realized that the magic "vaccinia" is a pathogen that can immunize them against diseases. Featuring the reduced virulence of a pathogen compared with that leading to diseases in humans, it can stimulate the body to develop a defense response to pathogens without causing sickness or severe sickness in the human body because of infection with such pathogen, based on which scientists were encouraged to think about the idea of the "attenuated vaccine," which can artificially weaken the virulence of human pathogens and help humans to obtain protective immunity.

The most typical attenuated vaccine is the rabies vaccine developed by a French microbiologist, Louis Pasteur.

Rabies is an extremely deadly zoonotic disease caused by rabies virus, which parasitizes dogs, bats, and rodents. Humans can be infected by a bite from the animal carrying the virus, which travels through the wound to the nervous system such as the brain and spinal cord in the circulatory system. Therefore, people infected often have symptoms such as "fear of water" after rabies onset and suffer from extreme stress and fear in severe cases. Children are the most susceptible to rabies infection. Even in the 21st century, without treatment, the fatality rate of rabies is almost 100% after onset of symptoms.

Rabies is widespread across the world. Until the end of the 19th century, Pasteur, who was determined to develop the rabies vaccine, obtained the pathogenic fluid from the brain marrow of the infected rabies and saliva to infect healthy rabbits, and collected the pathogenic fluid from rabbits with illness onset to continue to infect healthy rabbits. Through over 100 generations of the artificial culture of rabies pathogens, infected rabies brain marrow tissues were taken out and dried. Eventually, by grinding and dissolving the dried brain tissues, the first rabies vaccine was developed in human history.

Under technological conditions at that time, people did not know the existence of viruses, let alone realize their special biological nature. Pasteur mainly used multiple generations and drying methods in the

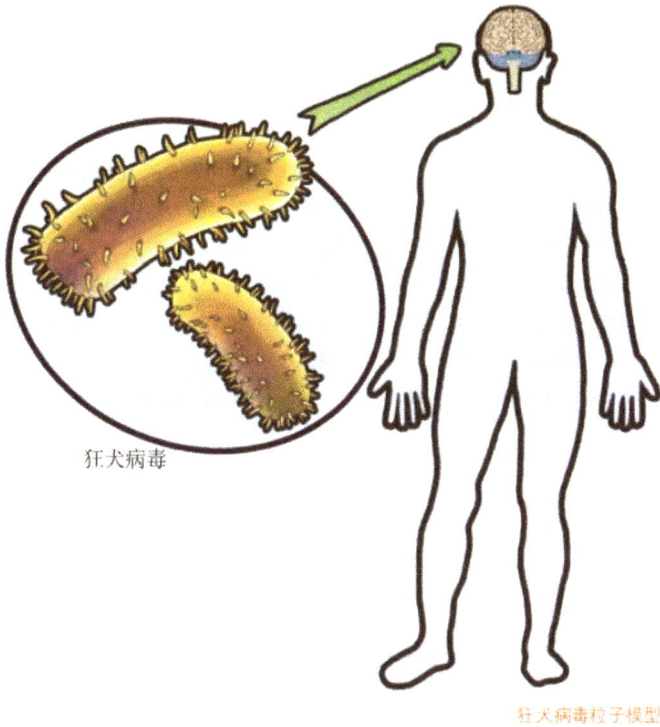

狂犬病毒

狂犬病毒粒子模型

Rabies Virus Particle Model

development of the rabies vaccine. On the one hand, multiple generations in the sound artificial environment gradually degenerated the species competition of the natural rabies virus; on the other hand, in the absence of water, the "source of life," the dry environment reduced the vitality and toxicity of the rabies virus; it was based on the success of vaccinia vaccine and the proposal of the theory of germ leading to diseases that Pasteur developed rabies vaccine, which became a milestone in the classical artificial development of "attenuated vaccines."

Inspired by the above idea, Bacillus Calmette–Guerin vaccine (BCG vaccine), the first vaccination administered to newborns, was a "marathon" achievement of "attenuated vaccines." In the beginning of the 20th century, French scientists Albert Calmette and Camille Guerin isolated *Mycobacterium bovis* from milk of cattle with tuberculosis and grew it in a beef bile–glycerine medium. With 13 years of continuous replanting of the culture in this medium (230 times), a safe and effective *Mycobacterium tuberculosis* attenuated strain was eventually obtained and the BCG vaccine was developed.

A live attenuated vaccine refers to the one that decreases virulence but maintains antigenicity after the processing of the pathogen. It remains a live virus which can induce a strong and long-lasting specific immune response without causing disease in the body. At present, live attenuated vaccines used in clinic include measles vaccine, chickenpox vaccine, encephalitis vaccine, polio vaccine, rabies vaccine, etc.

The general characteristic of these vaccines is: "attenuated" but "strong."

Inactivated Vaccines

At the end of the 19th century and beginning of the 20th century, in the development of attenuated vaccines, scientists gradually found that some microbes were difficult to be attenuated, some lost potential for vaccine development with the weakened virulence and following weak immuogenicity, and in some worse cases, contrary to the expectations, safety problems occurred with the reversion to a virulent organism in the body.

Based on above problems, vaccine development turned to another direction, namely, the inactivated vaccine.

In 1883, during the cholera epidemic in Egypt, scientists first identified the pathogenic bacterium causing cholera: *Vibrio cholerae*. In the following year, during the cholera epidemic in Spain, *Vibrio cholerae* isolates were attenuated and cultured, which were accordingly developed into the cholera attenuated vaccine. However, the vaccine always caused severe vaccine reactions and even deaths due to poor production conditions and underdeveloped technologies. Since then, though many attempts have been made to improve the attenuated vaccine and produce the inactivated vaccine, results were not satisfactory.

In 1896, a German scientist Wilhelm Kolle developed the inactivated cholera vaccine from cholera broth cultures heated at 56°C for an hour with carbolic acid for anticorrosion. When used by the Romanian army during the Balkan War in the 1920s, the vaccine was reported to have the desirable immune effect only second to vaccinia and rabies vaccines. During World War I, the vaccine was used by all countries involved and desirable immune results were achieved. Improved vaccines, which were used by German and Austrian armies, increased the immune protection effect.

In 1897, Waldemar Haffkine, a Ukrainian scientist, developed the inactivated plague vaccine from *Yersinia pestis* heated at 70°C for an hour. Desirable preventive effects were achieved when it was extensively inoculated in the plague outbreak in Bombay, India. After the success of this method, many countries around the world developed inactivated plague vaccines, which were widely and safely inoculated on the population across the world to effectively make them immune against plague.

In 1937, when the culprit of the influenza pandemic in World War I was identified, US troops hoped a safe and effective flu vaccine could be designed. Jonas Salk and Thomas Francis developed an inactivated influenza virus within two years, which not only achieved desirable clinical and commercial results, but also played an important role in controlling influenza outbreaks in America after World War II. In 1954, by means of inactivating the cultured poliomyelitis strain with formaldehyde and maintaining its viral immunogenicity, Salk developed the inactivated polio vaccine, which successfully prevented poliomyelitis.

Inactivated vaccines are complete viruses or bacteria or their fragments which are first cultured and then inactivated with heat or chemical methods so that people inoculated could produce humoral immune responses. At present, inactivated vaccines mainly include diphtheria vaccine, influenza vaccine, rabies vaccine, etc.

The general characteristic of inactivated vaccines is "safe" and "effective."

Subunit Vaccines

With the development of molecular biology technology, a specific antigen extracted from viruses or bacteria, which are the main components of vaccines, can be used to trigger a specific immune response in the body. This idea contributed to the birth of subunit vaccines.

Hepatitis B vaccine, which is designed for the prevention of major infectious diseases of viral hepatitis, is a typical subunit vaccine.

At present, there are more than 240 million people suffering from chronic liver infections in the world. In China, around 90 million people are infected with hepatitis B virus, which will cause a persistent infectious disease, leading to a high mortality rate due to liver cirrhosis and liver cancer.

In 1963, an abnormal antigen was identified in the serum of an Australian patient and was named Australian antigen (Aa). In 1967, the antigen was proved to be associated with hepatitis B virus and was renamed HBsAg, namely, hepatitis B surface antigen. It was not until in 1970 that the structure of hepatitis B virus was observed under an electron microscope.

Scientists immediately started exploring a vaccine for hepatitis B virus. In 1971, based on the idea of designing a subunit vaccine, the effective live surface antigen was extracted from isolated and purified plasma of asymptomatic hepatitis B carriers. This antigen was then developed to the first hepatitis B vaccine, which was also known as "plasma-derived vaccine" since it was derived from human plasma.

This subunit vaccine was soon produced and used for disease prevention due to the good immunogenicity and reactivity of hepatitis B surface antigen. However, the production of hepatitis B vaccine is based on plasma from hepatitis B patients, which raises people's concerns about the safety of plasma products since hepatitis B patients are also at high risks of other diseases. Considering the limited source, production cost, and plasma safety of plasma-derived vaccine, new molecular biology technologies provide novel methods and techniques for subunit vaccine development.

The corresponding protein can be finally encoded according to the genetic information of nucleic acid DNA through genetic engineering. In fact, the hepatitis B virus surface antigen extracted from plasma is also a protein. If the DNA code of the surface antigen could be decoded and the corresponding active protein could be expressed by engineered microorganisms, the specific immunity against hepatitis B virus can be induced in the body without virus culture or safety risks of plasma.

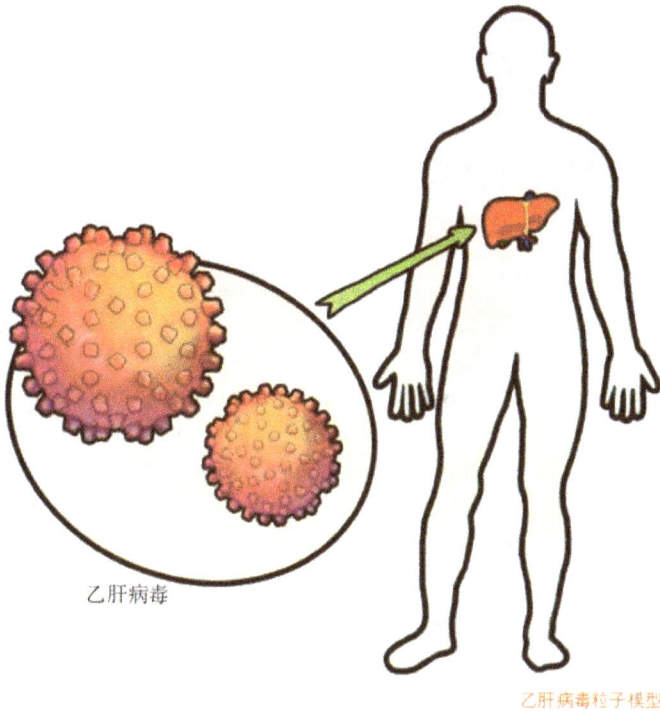

乙肝病毒

乙肝病毒粒子模型

Hepatitis B Virus
Hepatitis B Virus Particle Model

Therefore, in 1979, the American scientist William Rutter cloned the DNA molecular sequence encoded on the hepatitis B virus surface antigen into the protein expression system of *Escherichia coli* through recombinant DNA technology. Modified engineered bacterial carriers can express and produce large numbers of hepatitis B virus surface antigens. In 1982, through further optimization, the hepatitis B virus surface antigen could also be expressed in engineered yeast cells and was confirmed to have protective immunity in orangutans. In 1986, this type of hepatitis B subunit vaccine was developed and approved for clinical use.

Subunit vaccine is a vaccine that induces a protective immune response in the body by making use of some immunogenic proteins of microorganisms. The "plasma-derived vaccine" and genetically engineered vaccine for hepatitis B prevention are subunits of complete hepatitis B virus antigens extracted from plasma or isolated and expressed from genetically engineered microorganisms. Therefore, they are also known as subunit vaccines.

The general characteristics of subunit vaccines are "safe" and "specific."

Virus-like Particle Vaccines

Virus-like particles are molecules that closely resemble viruses, but are non-infectious because they contain no viral genetic material.

There are three different types of hepatitis B virus particles under an electron microscope, including small spherical particles, tubular particles, and large spherical particles. Among them, the large spherical particle, with core and envelope, is a complete hepatitis B virion composed of DNA, HBsAg, and enzyme protein. The small spherical particle, composed of enveloped proteins, contains no viral genomes. The tubular particle is composed of small spherical particles in series. Both the small spherical particle and tubular particle are known as subviral particles.

Virus-like particles can be regarded as an "alternative" manifestation of inactivated or subunit vaccines since they are composed of antigenic protein particles and contains no nucleic acid components that guide viral infection and replication.

With the same spatial structure as natural viruses, virus-like particles can intensively display antigen epitopes. Thus, strong immune response can be triggered in the body. Virus-like particle vaccines generally have stronger immunogenicity than subunit vaccines and recombinant protein vaccines, which can stimulate not only humoral immune response, but also cellular and mucosal immunity, making them the promising candidate vaccine or vector.

Structural proteins in human and animal viruses such as HIV, HBV, and HPV can be automatically assembled as virus-like particles in the host expression system, including mammalian cell expression system, insect cell expression system, *E. coli*, and yeast expression system.

HPV, which can infect epidermises and mucosal tissues in human body, was first observed under an electron microscope in 1949. It was

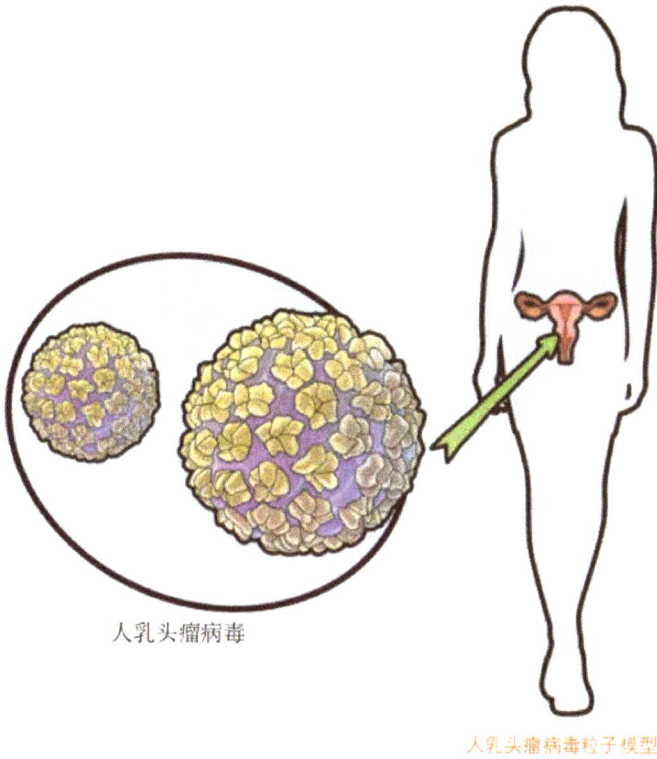

人乳头瘤病毒

人乳头瘤病毒粒子模型

Human Papillomavirus
Human Papillomavirus Particle Model

initially thought to be associated with skin papules and warts. It was not until in 1991 that a large-scale epidemiological investigation confirmed HPV as the causative agent of cervical cancer.

Around 500,000 women are diagnosed with cervical cancer worldwide and 288,000 women die from the diseases. There are over 100 varieties of HPV, which can be classified as high-risk and low-risk HPV types based on their different pathogenicity. There are 15 high-risk strains of HPV that can lead to cervical intraepithelial neoplasia and cervical cancer.

The HPV vaccine is a cancer vaccine that is composed of self-assembling, virus-like particles of the surface protein L1 of HPV. In 2006, HPV vaccine was approved by the US Food and Drug Administration.

At present, there are 2-valent HPV vaccine, 4-valent HPV vaccine, and 9-valent HPV vaccine. These vaccines targeting high-risk HPV types can prevent different HPV types: a 2-valent HPV vaccine can protect against HPV types 16 and 18; a 4-valent HPV vaccine can protect against HPV types 6, 11, 16, and 18; a 9-valent HPV vaccine can protect against HPV types 6, 11, 18, 31, 33, 45, 52, and 58.

More monitoring and data need to be accumulated although 12 years have passed since the invention of the HPV vaccine. At least so far, it is very effective in preventing cervical cancer. We should remain keeping alert in preventing HPV-related diseases since there are 100 HPV types while current vaccines only target high-risk HPV type.

The general characteristics of virus-like particle vaccines are "effective" and "safe."

There are six live attenuated vaccines and eight inactivated vaccines in China's vaccines of statutory immunization program (namely, officially-classified category 1 vaccines).

From Section 1, it can be seen that the vaccine design is based on the fundamental principle of immunity, while the research and development of vaccines vary from virus to virus.

In Section 2, let us explore inactivated influenza vaccines and influenza virus polyvalent vaccines.

Polyvalent vaccines predict the subtypes of influenza viruses that will be circulating based on the epidemiological surveillance and biological analysis. For example, 3-valent vaccine is a mixture of three possible cultured and inactivated virus subtypes. Polyvalent viral vaccines contain a variety of immune antigens.

2. Influenza Vaccine

Influenza viruses have short "lifetime," but are constantly mutating "from generation to generation." Their evolutionary characteristics help them to evade host immune surveillance and attack and allow new viruses to "run away."

Neutralizing antibodies are corresponding antibodies produced when the pathogenic microorganism invades the body, which can effectively produce protective immunity by binding to specific antigens and "neutralizing" biological functions of antigens. Accordingly, non-neutralizing antibodies are those that bind to but do not neutralize antigens.

Viral neutralizing antibodies mainly target the surface glycoprotein hemagglutinin, or HA. Thus, the HA mutation is an important "magic weapon" for the immune evasion of influenza viruses, and other genetic mutations also play an auxiliary role in the viruses' escape from attack. The main physiological defense mechanism against attack is the acquired immune system induced by viruses either through natural infection or active vaccination.

Among immunoglobulin subtypes of the neutralizing antibody, IgA and IgG are the main hemagglutinin directly defending against the surface of the virus: IgA secretes in the mucosal surface of the respiratory tract and neutralizes influenza viruses, and IgG circulates in the blood and penetrates the respiratory tract and lungs. Immunoglobulin neutralizes the virus by binding to the hemagglutinin receptor site to prevent the virion from attaching and entering the cell, or by binding to other parts of the hemagglutinin or neuraminidase to affect their functions. However, the mutated influenza virus can evade the "Dharma eye" of the antibody due to the misjudgment of "locking" the attacking target of the immune response, which is caused by the changed "physical evidence" in the viral antigen epitopes "collected" by B lymphocytes.

Therefore, it is necessary to update influenza vaccines "generation after generation" each year to fight potential epidemics of primary strains of influenza A virus (H1N1 and H3N2) and Victoria and Yamagata lineages of influenza B virus. Even though antibodies to the virus might have been produced in the body before, they may not be able to fight the predominant circulating flu strain.

So, What is the Mysterious "Virus Prediction Organization"?

In 1947, WHO established the Global Influenza Surveillance Network responsible for monitoring the latest circulating influenza virus strains to determine subunit flu vaccines. By June 2018, there were 144 National Influenza Centers (NICs) in 114 countries, 5 Core Laboratories for Vaccine

Regulation; 5 WHO Collaborating Centers for Reference and Research on Influenza in the UK, US, Australia, Japan, and China; and 1 WHO Collaborating Center for Studies on the Ecology of Influenza in Animals.

All the regions worldwide are taking initiative in strengthening capacities of detection and surveillance of novel influenza viruses and sharing of virus resources and information. The WHO Member States are grouped into 6 regions with 6 regional offices responsible for 43 major countries, including African Region, Region of the Americas, Eastern Mediterranean Region, European Region, South-East Asia Region, and Western Pacific Region.

Sharing of virus resources and information has been conducted through WHO's Global Influenza Surveillance and Response System (GISRS). Considering "antigenic shift" and "antigenic drift" caused by influenza virus mutation, the global sharing of virus strain resources can better deal with the uncertainty of virus epidemic and ensure the strategic reserve of vaccine strain "library." GISRS is a system committed to seasonal risk assessment, virus identification, development of candidate vaccine viruses, reagents and diagnostics, and recommendations of vaccine strains for seasonal influenza vaccines.

It is necessary to match flu vaccine compositions with seasonal predominant strains in order to "launch a precise attack."

At present, recommendations for three influenza vaccine strains are formulated by WHO based on the large-scale epidemiological data, identification of viral antigens, and genetic evolution analysis to run the Influenza Surveillance and Vaccine Recommendation Systems. To improve the efficiency of influenza vaccine in preventing epidemic strains every year, the WHO proposed to develop a trivalent influenza vaccine on the basis of the surveillance of global novel influenza virus strains by selecting two influenza A strains and one influenza B strain of the influenza vaccine according to annual predictions of "seasonally prevalent" virus. However, more recently, quadrivalent vaccines have been developed which contain two influenza B strains (Yamagata and Victoria lineages).

For example, from 1987 to 1997 influenza seasons, three virus strains were fully matched with the prevalent ones in five years. Despite uncertain virus mutations leading to occasional inconsistency with vaccine viral strains and reduced protective efficacy, it remains a very effective influenza prevention and control system for global health macro-strategies. We can neither deny the general trend of predicted vaccines for virus prevention nor refuse to inoculate vaccines due to concerns of risks just because of the occurrence of an opportunistic event.

The efficacy of the monovalent vaccine is often critical in vaccine production. Since influenza vaccine is a "trivalent vaccine" system containing three viral strains, the efficacy of each monovalent vaccine will be synthesized in an influenza vaccine against three predicted epidemic strains. In general, when the first batch of trivalent vaccines are applied to the public, clinical serological studies in two groups will be conducted immediately to test and assess the protective efficacy and level. In many countries, a uniform standard of subunit vaccines has been established and vaccine immunogenicity standard began to be implemented.

Taking all these factors into consideration, the WHO issues its recommendations for influenza vaccine formulations in February and conducts a second review in September, providing formulations of seasonal influenza vaccine strains for northern and southern hemispheres during the respective winter seasons. Vaccine production is always in winter since it generally takes a six-month period to produce vaccines after the WHO's recommendations on vaccine strains.

Since the launch of the Global Action Plan for Influenza Vaccines, US$50 million has been invested by the WHO and US$1 billion has been contributed by many countries and other agencies to support influenza vaccine production. Currently, 300 million doses of vaccines are produced annually. The Global Action Plan for Influenza Vaccines is expected to expand production capacity for up to 1 billion doses of influenza vaccines for 2018 to 2019 influenza seasons.

How to Select Defense Weapons After Predicting Upcoming Attacks by Epidemic Viral Strains?

Most influenza vaccines in the world are inactivated ones with excellent safety records. Hundreds of millions of influenza reagents are distributed around the world every year with extremely rare reports on side effects. Moreover, influenza vaccination has been proved to be highly effective.

The original influenza inactivated vaccine, composed of whole inactivated virus subunits, has relatively high immunogenicity. However, despite improved virus purification technologies, local and systemic side effects may occur in the process of whole inactivated vaccination, especially in children and people with weak immune systems.

Later, the split-virion vaccine developed, and the inactivated virion could produce almost equal immunogenicity with few side effects compared to that of the whole-virus vaccine. Its disadvantage is the relatively low immunogenicity to individuals who are not exposed to the virus infection. Those people can obtain adequate protection via strengthening their immunity, thus making the split-virion inactivated vaccine the most widely used influenza vaccine.

The subunit vaccine extends the theory of antigens. Hemagglutinin and neuraminidase, which are influenza virus surface antigens of subunit vaccines, are components of viral particles obtained through isolation and purification. Subunit vaccines can cause minimum local and systemic side effects compared to whole-virus inactivated vaccines and split-virion inactivated vaccines. As the major virus surface proteins in inducing the production of neutralizing antibodies, the hemagglutinin and neuraminidase in subunit vaccines can produce relatively good immunogenicity, which provides another path for vaccine research and development. The latest influenza subunit vaccines also include hemagglutinin vaccines produced in large quantities in in vitro expression systems.

The Production of Inactivated Vaccines Requires the Virus Culture, which has Two Key Elements: Quantity and Quality

Recommended virus strains predicted to circulate are usually cultured in chicken embryos. At present, almost all influenza vaccines are produced in chicken embryo culture, since strains identified by WHO can grow well in the host, replicate well in chicken embryos, and carry the recommended hemagglutinin and neuraminidase. As an old Chinese saying goes, "Food and fodder should go ahead of troops and horses." Prior to the start of the vaccine manufacturing cycle every year, vaccine manufacturers must first make "chicken embryo budget," order sufficient amounts of chicken embryos, and produce influenza vaccine strains after the WHO issues recommendations on vaccines and their formulations.

Vaccine contraindications include egg allergy and a history of allergy to vaccines. Allergic reactions are mostly resulted in egg-derived ingredients in the vaccine, especially ovalbumin. Nevertheless, these problems may be avoided through the cell culture technique applied in the production of influenza vaccines.

MDCK cells, the main in vitro hosts of influenza viruses, can be used for cultures of inactivated viruses and subunit vaccine strains, which have similar antigenicity to that of vaccines cultured in chicken embryos. Instead of relying on the supply of chicken eggs, cell culture strains make vaccine production more flexible, which is even more important in the avian influenza epidemic outbreak since the possible supply failure of eggs can turn the "fodder" to "enemy resources."

Up to now, the indicator to show the efficacy of influenza vaccines has always been the appropriate level of virus-neutralizing antibodies induced in serum. These antibodies mainly target envelope glycoproteins of viruses — hemagglutinin and neuraminidase — among which hemagglutinin is the main target of virus-neutralizing antibody. It has been proved that hemagglutinin can penetrate from the blood to lungs through the circulatory system, preventing severe viral pneumonia.

Therefore, the efficacy of vaccines is assessed based on serologic data, particularly antibody titers and serum protection rates. Hemagglutination inhibition (HI) activity is a common method of detecting antibody titers, in which agglutination of red blood cells (RBCs) will be caused by the attachment of sialic acid receptors on the surface of RBCs to hemagglutinin of influenza virus, HI will be titrated by a series of dilutions of antibodies, and the HI titer of the antibody will be determined by the highest dilution when hemagglutination is completely inhibited.

At present, the standard dose for the trivalent influenza vaccine candidate is 15 micrograms per viral strain, which can induce protective neutralizing antibodies sufficient for the immune system to prevent influenza virus.

Humans often hope everything perfect in their pursuit of happiness. There are "trivalent," "quadrivalent," and "polyvalent" influenza vaccines. "Polyvalent" is by no means "full valent." What kind of "valent" is a "perfect valent"? This is a question.

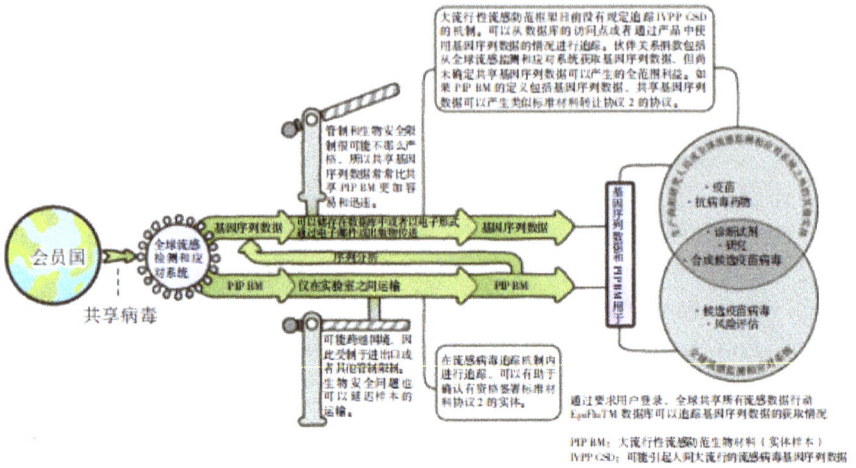

世界卫生组织大流行性流感防范框架下共享的实体样本和基因序列数据

Member countries

Virus sharing

Global Influenza Surveillance and Response System

Genetic sequence data

PIP BM

Regulation and biosecurity restrictions may be not so strict that it is often much easier and faster to share genetic sequence data than PIP BM.

It can be stored in a database or disseminated electronically via E-mail or publications

Sequence analysis

It can only be transmitted between laboratories

Influenza virus samples, which may be transmitted across national borders, are subject to import, export, or other regulatory restrictions. Biosafety issues may also result in the delay of sample shipment.

There is no restriction on the mechanism for tracing IVPP GSD in the Pandemic Influenza Preparedness Framework. IVPP GSD can be traced by visiting the access point of database or analyzing the genetic sequence data used in products. Partnership contributions contain the access to genetic sequence data from the GISRS. However, the full scope of benefits from sharing genetic sequence data remains unidentified. If the definition of PIP BM covers genetic sequence data, its sharing can lead to a protocol similar to Standard Material Transfer Protocol 2.

Genetic sequence data

PIP BM

Tracing based on the influenza virus tracking mechanism can facilitate the identification of entities eligible to sign Standard Material Protocol 2.

Gene sequence data and PIP BM can be used for

Vaccines

Antiviral drugs

Diagnostic reagents

Research

Synthesis of candidate vaccine viruses

Candidate vaccine viruses

Risk assessment

Users are required to log in and join the global sharing influenza data actions

EpiFluTM database can trace the access to genetic sequence data

PIP BM: Pandemic Influenza Preparedness Biomaterials (physical samples)

IVPP GSD: Genetic Sequence Data from Influenza Viruses with Human Pandemic Potential (IVPP GSD)

Physical Samples and Genetic Sequence Data Sharing under the WHO Pandemic Influenza Preparedness Framework

Everyone hopes that the polyvalent vaccine against viruses can "make the right prediction for the upcoming virus." However, it remains possible to "make wrong predictions" since predictive models are based on existing data. It is due to the high mutation rate, rapid transmission, and susceptible pathogenicity of influenza virus that the whole world will be committed to developing a broad-spectrum influenza virus vaccine featuring long protection period and desirable immune efficacy targeting a wide range of virus subtypes.

3. Universal Influenza Vaccine

Influenza, which has resulted in four pandemics within two centuries and launched seasonal attacks almost every year, continues to mutate and always causes dangerous symptom, causing 250,000 to 500,000 deaths worldwide every year.

An "ultimate goal" will be the development of a universal influenza vaccine based on a broad array of virus strains against which it can generate protection. There are a series of stage goals before achieving the ultimate goal. For example, the single-strain vaccine is designed to protect against a specific virus strain; the subtype virus vaccine is designed to protect against a specific subtype virus; the broad-spectrum influenza vaccine can protect against multiple virus subtypes; the generic influenza vaccine can protect all viruses of group one or group two. The protection efficacy of influenza vaccines is usually between 10% and 60% due to virus mutations and wrong predictions of vaccine strains. Moreover, the subunit strains of the influenza vaccine must be updated every year to protect against a seasonal new flu strain.

Before achieving the "ultimate goal," the National Institutes of Health held a thematic forum on the development of a universal influenza vaccine in 2017 to propose development goals and strategies in the future, and achieve the "limited goal" of a universal vaccine: with the protective efficacy of 75% lasting over 12 months for group 1 or 2 influenza A virus in all populations.

	疫苗	保护范围
	毒株特异性	病毒流行株
	亚型特异性	单一血凝素亚型（如 H1）
	多亚型	单一组多血凝素亚型（如 H1/H5/H9）
	泛组	覆盖所有 1 组或 2 组
普适性	通用流感疫苗	全部甲型流感（+/− 乙型流感）

美国国立卫生研究院：通用流感疫苗发展策略

Universality

Vaccine

Strain-specific

Subtype-specific

Multi-subtypes

Pan-group

Universal influenza vaccine

Coverage

Current circulating strains

All strains within a single hemagglutinin subtype (e.g., H1)

Multiple Hemagglutinin subtypes within single group (e.g., H1/H5/H9)

Covering all group 1 or 2

All influenza A (+/− influenza B)

NIH: Strategy for Developing a Universal Influenza Vaccine

The scientific research directions will be systematically laid out in three main areas including viral epidemiology, immunology, and vaccine design as well as related resources and technical support fields, so as to achieve the stage goal of developing a universal influenza vaccine which can generate a sustainable protection against a variety of influenza strains and upcoming prevalent virus strains.

"Three Questions": Virus, Immune Function, Vaccine Design

The protective efficacy of vaccines will be directly influenced by the research on transmission, epidemiology, and pathogenesis of influenza viruses during vaccine research and development. More accurate predictions of vaccine strain subunits can be generated for populations immunized by the flu vaccine in different areas according to the research on relations between virus prevalence and clinical pathogenesis, interactions between disease prevalence and environmental factors, and the clinical pathogenic mechanism of severe patients, infants, and the elderly attacked by seasonal influenza, as well as the antigen monitoring and comparative analysis of influenza virus infection between animals and humans. These more accurate predictions contribute to strategies for the development of improved vaccines in vaccinated populations and the warning and response to the novel virus strains that may mutate.

The key to answering the question of protective efficacy in humans is to study the immunity to influenza virus and the protective immune function in humans. The study on protective agents of the immune system in humans naturally infected or immunized will provide better strategies for the protection of novel influenza strain vaccines under pre-immunization conditions; vaccine-induced innate and acquired immune response to viruses will activate and strengthen the antiviral effects of humoral and cellular immunity, whereas the research and development of standard and uniform diagnostic and test standards and vaccine technology platforms will facilitate the establishment of the efficacy evaluation and design support system on the basis of novel standard vaccines.

Based on new scientific ideas and technologies, breakthrough will be achieved in the rational design of a universal influenza vaccine, including designing vaccine-functional antigens such as viral hemagglutinin non-surface unfolded antigen, neuraminidase, M2 ion channel, and nuclear protein; designing specific vaccine adjuvants that enhance immune response, protection period, and range; and designing a clinical trial platform system for novel vaccines, adjuvants, and vaccination systems, all of which will make it possible to discover the stable and long-term protective effect against a wide range of influenza viruses, to develop the novel antigen or adjuvant combinations that identify and induce long-term protective effects in human body against a wide range of viruses, and create the clinical trial condition and environment for the research, development, and assessment of the next-generation influenza vaccine.

In addition to the "three problems," the "four establishments" will be briefed.

"Four Establishments:" Establish Animal Models, Monitor Mechanisms, Immune Standards, and Prediction Systems

It is important to establish animal models essential for vaccine development since there is no single animal model that can fully recapitulate human diseases. Epidemiological and immune response monitoring systems are established for individual groups to verify and optimize vaccine designs since individuals will acquire disparate immunities by being exposed to different influenza viruses or vaccinations. The establishment of a human health immune clinical system is the standard which can best demonstrate the vaccine efficacy in virus infection and immunity As an interdisciplinary field, systems biology is the study to establish resource and information systems in big data analysis, which will improve the capacity of influenza prediction and vaccine design.

The plan is expected to be executed in the future. Now let us talk about the present and "crossing a river by feeling our way over the stones."

The Hemagglutinin that is "Hard to Guess"

The hemagglutinin remains undoubtedly the first vaccine component to be studied. Hemagglutinin, the skeleton of a universal vaccine, can induce highly desirable immunogenicity response in human body, making it the "chief protein" in the universal influenza vaccine design.

In 2013, scientists in Maryland Vaccine Research Center in the US developed a general vaccine against major influenza viruses, which can induce broad-spectrum antibodies in mice by fusing the influenza virus hemagglutinin protein antigens with the ferrous ion transporter in the blood to neutralize most influenza viruses and even prevent virus mutations yet to come. As the animal model susceptible to influenza viruses, ferrets injected with the general vaccine have been further showed to protect against all influenza viruses emerging and circulating from 1934 to 2007.

In 2015, two research teams in the US used the H1N1 influenza virus hemagglutinin protein as the skeleton to obtain recombinant hemagglutinin substrate protein through recombinant DNA technology and constructed a macromolecule particle made of 24 ferrous ion proteins enveloping 8 hemagglutinin proteins by self-assembling the hemagglutinin substrate protein with a ferrous ion protein.

The two teams used H5N1 influenza virus to test the "broad spectrum" function of the two vaccine candidates, respectively. It was found that in the animal experiment, the vaccine produced high antibody levels and achieved desirable protective effect in animals, which was an important outcome in developing a universal influenza vaccine.

In 2018, a new study from Georgia State University in the US showed that researchers had developed a nano-universal vaccine against influenza A virus, which was based on the hemagglutinin substrate with a highly conserved protein domain. Producing long-lasting immunity in mice, the vaccine can break the limitations of existing seasonal influenza vaccines to fully protect them from various influenza A viruses.

The vaccine is a nano-particle packaging protein substrate as a double-layered protein. The mice were inoculated twice through intramuscular injection and then exposed to H1N1, H3N2, H5N1, and H7N9 influenza viruses, the results of which showed that the vaccine provided universal and full immune protection against the lethal influenza virus and significantly reduced the virus amount in lungs of mice.

In the future, further clinical trials remain necessary for testing the timeliness and durability of vaccine-induced immunity in humans.

Multi-gene "Massive Defensive Weapons"

Among many types of RNA, microRNA/miRNA is a single-stranded RNA molecule in the cell that is 21–25 nucleotides in length. It is not involved in protein coding but can regulate gene expression and protein function. It is due to its small size that miRNA is always used as a "genetic tool" in molecular biology.

In 2015, new progress in influenza vaccine research was made by research teams from CAS, which proved that miRNA, the conserved fragments of targeting influenza virus, can be used as a new approach to influenza prevention and control. It was found that vaccinated mice were 100% protected against homologous H1N1 subtype influenza virus and 40%–100% protected against heterologous H5N1 and H9N2 subtypes influenza viruses.

Through software design and in vitro cell screening, team members obtained seven miRNAs with effective antiviral effect targeting influenza virus conserved genes such as NP, M1, and M2, and seven influenza vaccines with different influenza-specific miRNA by cloning the screened miRNA into adenoviral vectors. It is expected to be further developed into a new broad-spectrum universal flu vaccine.

"Unusual" Cellular Immunity

As the main force of antiviral infection immunity, immune cells can differentiate into T-killer cells to eliminate infected host cells or helper T cells to release cytokines to regulate vascular permeability, activate macrophages, remove invasions of foreign pathogens in the body, and collaborate with the humoral immune to release antibodies against viruses.

A series of peptides have been discovered by scientists based on the internal structure of influenza viruses. Several types of T cells can be produced in the immune system of the body and interact with influenza virus peptides that are presented by leukocyte antigens. The influenza vaccine, which was designed based on the peptide of conserved structure of virus, would activate immune responses of T cells, provide long-lasting immunity against a broad spectrum of influenza virus strains, and facilitate the development of a universal influenza vaccine.

To form peptide chains, amino acids are joined together by peptide bonds, and several peptide chains make up a protein through spatial structures with certain functions. Conserved peptides in internal structures of these viruses can be found in almost all influenza virus strains. So far, the vaccine only works well in specific virus trials, offering a possible prospect for a potential universal influenza vaccine.

In 2013, a research team in Imperial College London found that healthy volunteers had far more T cells than those infected with flu in the influenza season, since killer T cells can defend against nuclear proteins of the influenza virus. The nuclear protein of the influenza virus is stable, based on which a vaccine can be designed to activate T cells to rapidly proliferate in the body. It can effectively defend against major influenza viruses and greatly expand the effective scope of influenza prevention and control.

In 2014, a research team from the US found that, in the influenza pandemic, some elderly people had conserved T-cell epitope immune response to the novel influenza virus despite lacking the humoral immune response induced by B cells. By screening the conserved gene sequence of hemagglutinin and neuraminidase of H1N1 influenza virus, these conserved protein epitopes can be used for developing novel H1N1 influenza vaccines.

By analyzing sequences of over 5,000 HA and NA in genes of pandemic influenza viruses since 1980, researchers eventually selected conserved sequences of 13 Has and 14 Nas, which cover 84% combined epitopes of pandemic H1N1 influenza strains, with higher or equal immunogenicity compared to 95% epitopes of other viral strains, making it possible to be the potential subunit candidate for H1N1 subtype influenza vaccine and the genetic engineering system for a universal influenza vaccine against other influenza subtypes.

The "Broad Avenue" for Neutralizing Antibodies

Fighting in the first line of defense against viruses is the most direct way to assess the vaccine effect at any time. "Antibodies" are always the first flash in the forefront of vaccine design. Since the invention of vaccines, the primary method is to test neutralizing antibody levels and their efficacy, which, therefore, has become a hotspot of research on a universal influenza vaccine.

In 2009, by means of phage display technology, researchers at Harvard Medical School in the US discovered a group of human influenza virus neutralizing antibodies featuring extensive neutralizing activity, which can effectively bind to the conserved region of hemagglutinin substrate structure to prevent the fusion process of influenza viruses and cell membranes and to destroy their abilities to infect human cells, which is expected to develop into an effective human monoclonal antibody.

In 2011, British and Swiss scientists used X-ray crystallography technology to isolate a super antibody that can neutralize all influenza A viruses. It was found that laboratory mice and ferrets injected with the super antibody could be protected from viruses, including 16 subtypes from two large groups of influenza A virus, representing a critical milestone in the development of a universal influenza vaccine.

In 2011, American scientists discovered a neutralizing antibody called CH65 through medical screening, which could neutralize more than 30 influenza viruses to block them from invading human cells through heterologous binding to influenza virus hemagglutinin. Researchers will continue to study the selection of immune system for antibodies, providing clues to the search for a universal influenza vaccine.

In 2011, a research team from the US and the Netherlands discovered an antibody called CR8020, which was proved effective against H3 virus strain and H7 virus strain in an animal experiment. Before that, the team had discovered another antibody named CR6261, which was also proved in an animal experiment that the antibody could effectively defend against H1 virus strains, including H1N1, by blocking the infection of cells bound to conserved regions of the HA substrate. The combination of the above two antibodies is expected to develop a robust and long-lasting universal influenza vaccine.

In 2012, scientists obtained the antibody library from memory marrow cells in bone marrow samples from patients infected with the flu, and isolated a new antibody, C05, from the antibody library. C05, a monoclonal antibody of influenza A virus, can prevent virus infection in cell and mouse laboratories and can also be used to treat mice infected with influenza virus. With 100% effectiveness lasting for three days, the antibody was a great inspiration for designing a universal influenza vaccine as well as the antibody therapy.

Using X-ray crystallography, researchers found that antibody C05 bound to the influenza virus hemagglutinin receptor by avoiding highly variable regions and making use of a uniquely extended protein ring structure. The receptor binding domain was not significantly mutated among virus strains, allowing C05 to neutralize different subtypes of influenza A viruses in this unique way, including H1, H2, H3, and H9 subtypes.

C05 can bind to a particular region of hemagglutinin in such a precise way by highly intensive attaching its single ring structure to receptors. This approach is truly remarkable in addressing antigenicity and variability at the same time. However, while it is exciting to discover an antibody library built outside the body, it would be even more significant to design a universal antigen to stimulate human body to produce functional antibodies such as C05.

In 2012, a research team from the Netherlands and the US discovered the first human monoclonal antibody broadly protective against all influenza B viruses. With two previously discovered monoclonal antibodies capable of neutralizing group 1 and 2 influenza A virus, the discovery of the broad-spectrum monoclonal antibody against influenza B virus fills the gap of antibodies neutralizing against major influenza A and B viruses in humans, which is a critical step to the development of a universal influenza vaccine and antibody therapy.

The new research report confirms the activity of three monoclonal antibodies against human influenza B virus, of which CR9114 antibody successfully neutralizes influenza A and B viruses in the experiment of mice models. By identifying proteins in main regions where antibodies bind to the virus surface, it is possible to develop a universal vaccine based on CR9114 antibody–antigen design to provide long-term protection against all influenza A and B viruses and be used in immunotherapeutic medicine for influenza A virus.

In 2013, a research team from CAS developed a broadly neutralizing human monoclonal antibody against influenza A viruses in response to the H1N1 influenza pandemic in 2009. It was found that the neutralizing antibody can prevent viruses entering cells by inhibiting the fusion of virus hemagglutinin with human host cell membrane. The broad-spectrum neutralizing antibody can fight against a variety of influenza virus sub-types and the human monoclonal antibody is highly specific, both of which can be directly used in clinical medicine since they are highly safe to humans and cannot be attacked by human immune system, offering significant reference to the research and development of therapeutic anti-body and the universal influenza vaccine.

The researchers obtained hemagglutinin-specific memory B cells from volunteers inoculated with H1N1 influenza virus vaccine and dis-covered human monoclonal antibodies by means of single-cell genetic cloning technology. The results showed that the antibody was capable of identifying antigen epitopes of hemagglutinin substrate. Seven antibodies obtained had the activity to neutralize different influenza virus subtypes such as H1, H3, H5, H7, and H9.

In 2015, scientists from China and South Korea jointly discovered a new human antibody which can neutralize several influenza virus sub-types in mice. Researchers isolated a potent antibody against H1N1 virus from immune cells obtained from recovered patients. The antibody worked by binding to two hemagglutinin monomers. The antibody could generate broad-spectrum protection for mice infected with influenza A virus from H1N1, H3N2, H5N1, and H7N9 virus subtypes, which may facilitate the exploration of new antiviral therapies.

Nucleic Acids of the Vaccine "Upstream"

The design concept of the nucleic acid vaccine should be demonstrated by the function of antigen proteins. Both DNA and RNA vaccines have the advantages of rapidity, precision, and highly-effective molecular biology technique of nucleic acid manipulation, as well as serving potential pro-tein vaccines "downstream" candidates.

In 2012, German scientists designed a piece of mRNA directly encod-ing the hemagglutinin protein of H1N1 influenza virus. By injecting syn-thetic mRNA into the skin of mice, researchers could use animal cells to produce hemagglutinin protein antigens. This elicited an immune response that later protected mice, ferrets, and pigs from infection with influenza viruses. It is expected to exert protective effect on humans as well.

Unlike DNA influenza vaccine design, in which DNA has to enter a cell's nucleus to read the genetic information and then transcribe it into RNA before it is translated into target proteins, the simple RNA vaccine can directly encode proteins outside the nucleus. In addition, the research team used genetic techniques to improve the stability of mRNA, which could be a precise and effective technique in vaccine development though it was not a universal influenza vaccine.

In 2013, researchers at the University of Arizona in the US designed and built a vaccine system, in which DNA vaccines, efficiently delivered to host cells by engineered bacterial vectors, can encode and express vaccine antigen proteins in host cells to induce the human body to generate specific antibodies and immune response. It is shown the DNA influenza vaccine is effective in mice. This technique will provide a platform for the rapid development of a broad-spectrum vaccine.

"Computing Model" Vaccines to Block Influenza Viruses

In the Information Age, many vaccine designs could be proposed by experimental data simulation. It also represents an "indirect prevention" approach to deduce the relationship between influenza virus infections and efficacy of human vaccines by establishing various computational models and combining scientific and clinical data.

In 2012, researchers at Princeton University in the US developed a novel vaccine that inhibits the mutation and transmission of influenza viruses by working on protein conserved regions of viruses. It can resist the viruses' attack and destruction of the immune system and made the influenza virus less virulent and harder to spread. They predicted that the vaccine would not only protect people from infection, but also ameliorate such flu-like symptoms as coughing and runny nose, which thereby reduces the possibilities of virus transmission.

The research team used computational models to combine clinical data of the vaccine with influenza virus evolutionary and epidemic models. Targeting multiple conserved functional subunits of influenza viruses, the efficacy of newly designed universal vaccine could be demonstrated by two influenza outbreak indicators, the epidemic and infectious potential. The viruses are unable to do much harm to humans even if they are likely to infect them.

In addition, the new vaccine is designed to prevent the evolution of influenza viruses by blocking their transmissions. The "universal" influenza vaccine will be jointly used with existing influenza vaccines. The evolution and transmission of viruses will be slowed down and reduced by existing vaccines, which can be used for a longer period before being replaced and the universal vaccine which will block influenza virus evolution and prevent it from spreading.

The Counterstrike of "Conservatives"

The Matrix-2 (M2) protein is the transmembrane protein of the influenza A virus. It is highly conserved in different subtypes of influenza A virus and can serve as a conserved target in a universal vaccine. Contrary to the potent "radical" hemagglutinin, it is more difficult to develop vaccines using M2 proteins as effective antigen subunits since M2 proteins have been hidden in the microcosmic time and space for a long time.

In 1999, Belgian scientists developed a vaccine infusing M2 proteins with HBV core proteins by enhancing the immunogenicity of the M2 proteins of influenza virus. By means of intraperitoneal and intranasal vaccination in mice, it was found that the vaccine protected mice from influenza viruses and contributed to virus elimination in mice lungs. The mice remained immune six months after the last immunization and the vaccine was predicted to provide protection against a broad-spectrum of influenza A virus strains.

In 2011, researchers in South Korea developed an oral vaccine with M2 proteins of influenza virus as the antigen that induce the immune response in mice lungs. M2 protein is highly conserved in different influenza viruses. Therefore, though the oral vaccine can prevent mice from a variety of influenza virus infections, including highly pathogenic H5 and H1 subtype viruses, it does not have the same preventive effect against different viruses, indicating its limited protection against virus infections.

In 2018, researchers from CAS successfully developed a novel broad-spectrum mucosal nanovaccine against influenza virus, which was based on self-assembling nanoparticles demonstrating conserved M2 protein epitopes of H1N1 influenza virus. The vaccine can induce strong humoral, cellular, and mucosal immune response through nasal immunization, making vaccination safer and more convenient. The vaccine completely protects against not only H1N1 influenza virus, but also H9N2 influenza virus, the research of which is expected to develop into a broad-spectrum influenza vaccine in the future.

Nucleic Acid and Protein "Act Simultaneously"

When the study of proteins suffers from the bottleneck in vaccine development, nucleic acid is used as the pioneer in vaccine development. This approach is often used as an "updated" approach for research and development in influenza virus vaccines and "extended" to other disease vaccines.

In 2010, scientists from NIH developed a universal influenza vaccine. Scientists successfully induced experimental mice, ferrets, and monkeys to generate antibodies to prevent against a variety of influenza virus strains by adopting the two-step vaccination, including DNA vaccines and inactivated or attenuated vaccines, which laid the foundation for the development of long-lasting vaccines against various influenza virus strains. Further assessment on its safety and immunity on humans will be conducted.

Both DNA and inactivated or attenuated vaccines target hemagglutinin or neuraminidase antigen of influenza viruses. DNA vaccines were first used to prime the body's immune system and inactivated or attenuated vaccines were then used to boost the immune effect. It was found that the "prime-boost" immune mode can induce the immune response in the hemagglutinin substrate conserved domain antigen of influenza virus. The mode is expected to become a novel approach for the development of a universal influenza vaccine.

Hypersensitive "Eight Vajrapanis"

In general, a universal influenza vaccine is often designed to target humoral or cellular immunity. However, designers blaze a trail this time by particularly targeting the interferon with more than one fighting teams "ambushing in all sides."

In 2018, Chinese and American scientists developed a novel "Hyper Interferon Sensitive (HIS)" influenza vaccine strain, which can boost the immune system to fight against influenza strains. It was shown in the animal experiment that the novel vaccine could be safe and effective in inducing strong immune response in animals. The achievement, giving the new strategy for designing the next-generation virus vaccine, was expected to be developed into a universal influenza vaccine.

Interferon is a protein secreted by the host cell that can prevent against virus and regulate immune reactions. The influenza virus may be evolved to avoid interferon. By comparing and analyzing the relationship between the whole genome of influenza virus and interferon sensitivity, the research team proposed a systematic approach to vaccine development, incorporating eight interferon-sensitive influenza genes into a new influenza strain HIS.

The HIS virus is highly attenuated in the host cell, but it can induce interferon response, which generates continuous humoral and cellular immune response and provide protection against homologous and heterologous viruses. By lessening virus virulence and enhancing the immune response simultaneously, this approach can fight H1N1 and H3N2 subtypes of influenza virus strains and is expected to be widely applied in the development of vaccines against other pathogens.

We have crossed the river by feeling our way over many stones. However, they are just "drops in a bucket." Based on a wide range of research targets such as antigens, antibodies, fusion proteins, nanoparticles, or peptides, and using DNA, RNA, and even data simulations to conduct experiments, these designs are for the "possible upcoming day" of a universal influenza vaccine.

Hemagglutinin looks like a "small mushroom" under an electron microscope. The extended region of the surface antigen in the "mushroom head" serves as the primary region of antibody recognition and frequent variation. The existing inactivated vaccines are mainly composed of antigens from this region. When the basal "mushroom body" is covered by the "mushroom head," it will be difficult to extend its antigen region, leading

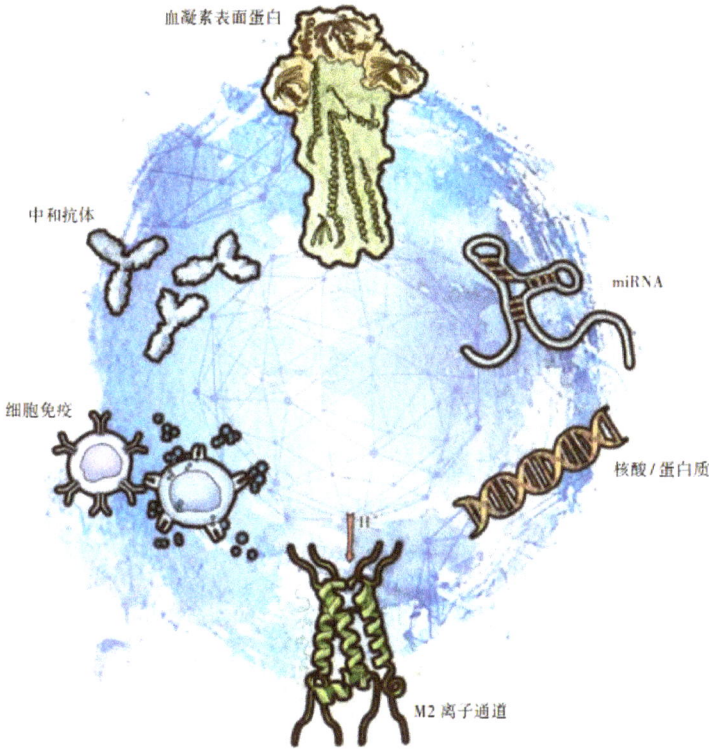

血凝素表面蛋白

中和抗体

miRNA

细胞免疫

核酸/蛋白质

M2 离子通道

通用流感疫苗设计理念

Hemagglutinin surface protein

Neutralizing antibody

Cellular immunity

M2 ion channel

Nucleic acid/ Protein

miRNA

Universal Influenza Vaccines Design

to low immunogenicity and antibody recognition, which means it is more conservative and difficult to mutate compared with the latter.

This can be difficult for "the little girl picking up the mushroom," the heroine in the Chinese song "A Little Girl with Mushrooms," who picks up mushrooms within her reach every year and also persists in picking those out of her reach.

How about extending antigens in the hemagglutinin substrate to be better recognized by immune cells so that they can generate better immune protection and obtain better broad-spectrum antiviral efficacy? However, after all, hemagglutinin is the active protein on the surface of virus. By means of protein crystallization imaging technology, it can be seen that hemagglutinin protein is composed of three protein monomers in the form of trimmer and the "little mushroom" is 13.5 nanometers in length with its "mushroom body" that is 7.6 nanometers long.

At this extreme micro scale, it is not so easy to "remove" the head from its body. A slight mistake may cause the loss of hemagglutinin activity and even the destruction in the protein structure, only leaving the molecular cloud "mushrooms."

Therefore, the above mistake may be made repeatedly until the day a universal vaccine is finally designed.

What are the new challenges we will face?

Chapter 10

A New Era

From "A"IV to "Z"IKV, humans have been constantly harassed by emerging and re-emerging viruses in these ceaseless "epidemic wars" without smoke. Novel viruses are continuously being discovered as they continue to mutate. Influenza viruses, coronaviruses, Ebola viruses, Zika viruses, and others are all armed with "fatal weapons" to aggressively attack humans and cause disease.

1. One Health

The year 2018 marks one-fifth of the new century. There is usually a flu season every year, and this year will be no exception. Flu outbreaks have been reported around the world, which remain to be a threat to the public health after the winter.

Influenza outbreaks were reported in all the US states in the same week by the Centers for Disease Control and Prevention for the first time in the last 15 years. In China, the number of reported flu cases tripled compared to flu seasons in the years immediately following the 2009 flu pandemic. It is also the second highest number of recorded flu cases in China, with many patients exhibiting severe clinical symptoms and even requiring hospitalization.

These facts should arouse our concern to rethink how to avoid another pandemic.

It can be found in surveillance data of reported cases in the world that influenza virus subtypes circulating in 2018 are complex, including influenza A virus subtypes H1N1 and H3N2, and influenza B Yamagata- and Victoria-lineage viruses. In the UK and US, influenza A virus subtype H3N2 is predominant, while in China, the circulating viruses are influenza A virus subtypes H1N1, H3N2 and influenza B Yamagata-lineage virus, and a few Victoria-lineage viruses. Vaccines have achieved only moderate protection although best efforts have been made across the world to predict the upcoming pandemic strain.

Since H5N1 avian influenza infections in humans occurred in 1997 in Hong Kong, China, human infection of different avian influenza virus subtypes has been reported now and then, with a high fatality rate of 30%–70%. It has been found that at least 15 influenza A viruses circulate in humans, including H1N1, H2N2, and H3N2. Among eight genes contained in the influenza A virus, there are "signs" of two additional HA and NA in bats apart from existing 16 HA and 9 NA. A simple calculation reveals that there are 144 different HxNy subtypes (excluding two novel influenza-like viruses in bats).

In nature, migrating birds travel thousands of miles in search of a landing place; in our life, the live bird trading practice facilitates the flying aerosol. For example, there are large numbers of poultry transportation and live poultry markets in East and Southeast Asia, which make us worried about the interspecies transmission of avian influenza to humans. The virus becomes more virulent and more easily transmitted once it is mutated, and its risk to humans will increase accordingly. At least in the system of disease prevention and control in our society, it is necessary to limit contact with live poultry, effectively cut off the route of virus transmission, and shift our efforts from behavior pattern change to health maintenance actions.

Influenza viruses are not alone. The coronavirus is a novel but familiar respiratory syndrome virus.

In 2003, the outbreak of SARS swept through major cities in China, causing great panic and anxiety. The severe acute respiratory disease caused by SARS coronavirus also facilitated China, the country with the largest population in the world, to establish a system for virus surveillance and disease prevention, which has gradually grown into an important cornerstone of its cooperation with WHO and other international organizations with continuous improvement in public health system.

In 2012, a novel MERS coronavirus re-emerged in the Middle East, causing human infections in Saudi Arabia and other regions. MERS-CoV infection cases were also reported globally, including imported coronavirus cases. In 2015, a MERS outbreak occurred in South Korea. A carrier of MERS-CoV was immediately detected and isolated upon entering the border of China. Further infections were prevented with a series of disease prevention and control measures. The surveillance and early warning system had ensured timely detection of the threat factor. Continuous progress was also achieved in the development of drugs and vaccines against the MERS-CoV. In 2018, MERS "visited" South Korea once again.

Ebola, one of the most dangerous viruses in the world, was first discovered in a river in an African village and named after it. It invaded the human world one more time, and this invasion occurred outside Africa.

The 2013–2015 Ebola outbreak in Western Africa affected many countries in Africa, Europe, and North America. The development of candidate vaccines against the virus were launched to effectively respond to the Ebola outbreak. Considering that the mutated virus strain might adversely affect the effectiveness of the vaccines, the full sequence of 175 viral genomes was used to confirm the mutation degree of Ebola virus and the current experimental vaccine was predicted to be effective. In addition, antiviral drugs were developed and used for disease treatment. For example, the ZMapp antibodies and vesicular stomatitis virus (VSV) and adenovirus (Ad5 and Ad3) vaccines played important roles in controlling the transmission of pathogens.

The Ebola epidemic was gradually brought under control within two years. However, the southern hemisphere was not in peace. South America, across the Atlantic Ocean from Africa, sounded an alert for Zika virus.

Though first discovered in 1947, Zika virus once again stirred tensions in the world since it could cause microcephaly, which would affect the next generations of hundreds of millions of families. Following small outbreaks in Micronesia in 2007 and Polynesia in 2013, the Zika virus epidemic occurred in Brazil in 2015 and 2016, and spread quickly to at least 84 countries and regions. Though a concerted global response quelled the Zika epidemic in November 2016, it would have a far-reaching negative impact.

In 2017, when Zika virus was not far away, yellow fever virus was imported by a worker returning from Angola to China during the Angola and Brazil outbreak. Meanwhile, Rift Valley Fever Virus (RVFV) was brought to China by a returning tourist. These events indicated that it would be increasingly difficult for humans to predict the next outbreak of emerging and re-emerging infectious diseases, as well as the identity, occurrence time, and location of pathogens.

People always neglect or forget the existence of emerging infectious agents such as SARS-CoV or MERS-CoV, re-emerging infectious agents like Ebola or Zika virus, and the potential variation and recombination of influenza viruses.

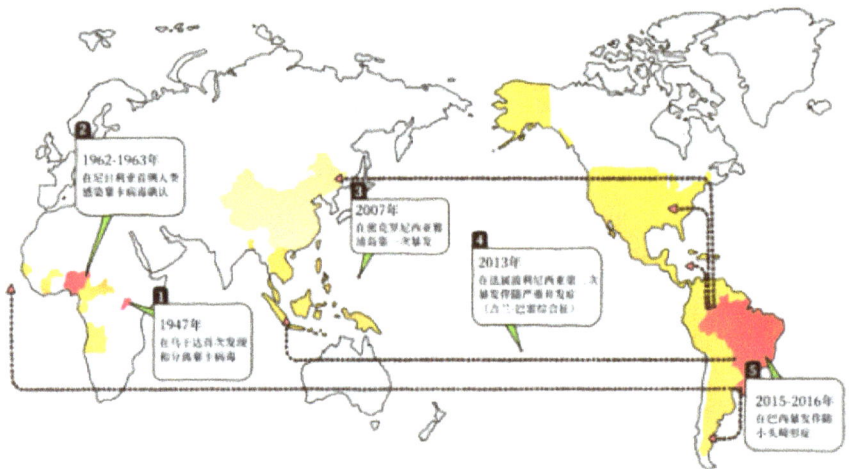

寨卡病毒在全球的流行和暴发

1. In 1947, Zika virus was first discovered and isolated in Uganda
2. From 1962 to 1963, the first human case was detected in Nigeria
3. In 2007, the first outbreak occurred in Micronesia Yap Island
4. In 2013, the second outbreak occurred in French Polynesia, causing severe complication, Guillain-Barre Syndrome
5. From 2015 to 2016, high incidents of microcephaly were reported in Brazil Outbreak and Prevalence of Zika Virus in the World

Globalization, urbanization, and climate change will make the future situation of disease prevention and control even more severe by affecting the pathogenicity, transmission, and host of pathogens. It is necessary for humans to further improve forward-looking strategies; understand the concept of "One health"; address human disease problems by focusing on protection of animal health and the development of ecological environment; and do more meticulous, thorough, and systematic work, such as upgrading pathogen monitoring system, developing antiviral drugs, and adopting effective measures for disease control. The modern disease treatment system is comprehensive, composed of scientists, clinicians, expert in public health, and nursing personnel. We are already capable of addressing challenges of existing pathogen spectrum diseases. It takes time and specific measures to overcome any challenge. Greater challenges are to be conquered in the future. We may face failure in this process, while we have to stand up and try to pursue success once again.

Transmissions of emerging and re-emerging infectious diseases pathogens know no national or geographic borders and require no visa for their "travel." With increasingly frequent international exchanges, prevention and control of diseases caused by pathogens has become a global responsibility. Therefore, cross-border international cooperation will become a trend in the future, which has begun to be put into practice.

The Global Virome Project will search for and discover unknown viruses around the world; the network of Centers for Disease Prevention and Control (CDCs) in Africa, which was established by the US CDC and Chinese CDC, will greatly improve the surveillance capacities around the world and better integrate itself into the global system for advancing the 21st century, the "big data" era; the Funding Project, launched by the World Bank, WHO, Japan, and Germany, will provide funds to developing countries against the risk of disease outbreak; the Coalition for Epidemic Preparedness Innovations (CEPI), Bill & Melinda Gates Foundation, Wellcome Trust, and the World Economic Forum will support vaccine development and its clinical applications.

Basic research is the living soul of scientific and technological innovation and a guide to public health policy and collaborative action on innovation. We should remember all these impressive facts, learn lessons from the past and present, and respond to the outbreak of a global pandemic by standing on the shoulders of giants to inspire the engines of a new era.

Knowledge is in every country the surest basis of public happiness.

–George Washington

According to traditional Chinese medicine, "sufficient healthy Qi inside the body will prevent invasion of pathogenic factors." The body's immunity and pathogenic factors are like the "white" and "black" game pieces. Progress in medicine, science, and technology is the basis for protecting human health. Disease prevention and control as well as scientific communication are the means to eliminating infections and diseases.

2. Science Popularization

There are two stones in the Olympic Village campus of CAS. One is from Mount Tai in China engraved "Still waters run deep," and the other is from Mount Fuji in Japan reading "Acquiring knowledge through probing into matters." These two stones commemorate the scientific and technological cooperation between China and Japan and also the whole world.

People ended up helplessly watching rampant diseases in World War I even if predictions and complete preparations for pandemics had been made. Any advance in medicine must first be scientifically proven to be effective before it can be used to fight against diseases. Science is neither a behavior nor a change, but a behavioral pattern or a cognitive accumulation. Science and technology constitute a primary productive force, which means it can never be obtained easily.

In 1900, it was more difficult to get into a respectable American college than into an American medical school. At least 100 US medical schools would accept any man willing to pay tuition; at most 20% of the schools required even a high school diploma for admission — much less any academic training in science — and only a single medical school required its students to have a college degree. Nor, once students entered, did American schools necessarily make up for any lack of scientific background. Many schools bestowed a medical degree upon students who simply attended lectures and passed examinations; in some, students never touched a single patient, and still obtained a medical degree.

Today, tremendous advances have been achieved in the field of medicine around the world. A student majoring in medicine must receive systematic science education courses, do internship in hospitals, obtain a series of medical certificates, and pass various assessment and examinations for doctors before he/she becomes qualified for a position in a medical institution. During this period, the development of natural science also gave birth to innovation in medicine. The research of natural science in medicine was gradually transformed into the study of medical problems in natural science.

Natural science faces a far greater challenge. Catching a cold is a good example. In clinical medicine, cold symptoms are often similar and its pathology also follows the development trend of respiratory diseases; further studies will show that factors causing cold are numerous and complicated, including the combination and mutations in various bacteria, the epidemic recombination or reassembly of disparate viruses, different immune responses, and functional pharmacology of vaccines and drugs. The seemingly macro-problem requires extremely detailed micro-solutions. People worldwide make joint efforts to "make great achievements" in the microbial world.

The road to science can never be smooth. Scientists have to endure loneliness and focus on research with a tranquil mind rather than simply chasing those superficial quantitative indicators or the so-called halo temptation. It is just like appreciating a famous painting when we were students. The teacher often told us the highlights of these paintings to help us understand these world-renowned paintings and even commented them with some obscure terminologies. Without extraordinary passion for art or cultivation in our family upbringing, we might be unable to understand how great the work was. However, when we occasionally see some paintings for beginners to appreciate, we will be reminded of excellent paintings of the same kind and associate them with those professional comments, which will evoke a strong sense of identity even if it cannot be expressed.

No matter how many centuries it has kept silent in those lonely nights, down-to-earth knowledge, like famous paintings, will no longer be a solitary lamp in the world of human cognition, but a brilliant treasure illuminating the human civilization.

The saying "Opportunity favors the prepared mind" is also the driving force for scientists devoted to research and enduring loneliness. There is a universally acknowledged causal relation in the logical principles: sufficient conditions and necessary conditions. The condition A is said to be sufficient for a condition B, if the truth of A guarantees the truth of B; the condition A is said to be necessary for a condition B, if the falsity of A guarantees the falsity of B. In our life and study, we always complain about "insufficient conditions" leading to our failure and believe we can accomplish something if we have sufficient conditions. However, in our lives, there are few things absolutely reaching the "sufficient conditions" since motion is eternal and rest is relative.

In times of hardship, when conditions exist, scientists went ahead; when they did not exist, they created them and went ahead. Only by making full use of existing and creating necessary conditions, can we finally achieve goals. "Making use of" and "creating" here belong to the connotation of sufficient conditions and contains conditions of "opportunity."

In the new era of fierce competition, when difficulties exist, people go ahead; when they do not exist, they create difficulties and go ahead, which is the optimistic attitude that motivates themselves. "Necessary condition" is universally acknowledged as a key factor of success, and to know oneself objectively and honestly is the basic requirement of this factor. Everyone has his own choices in life. We all have only 24 hours in a day, which means it is impossible for you to try everything.

It is found that 263 known viruses that have infected humans account for less than 0.1% of total numbers of suspected latent viruses that may infect humans. The most effective disease control requires first-class technology. In terms of H7N9, only by getting to its "bottom" can we know how far we have moved in our road to understanding the virus. To develop world-class science and technology, actions speak louder than words — as the adage goes "No sooner said than done."

Scientific progress and social development depend on four "Cs," namely Cooperation, Competition, Communication, and Coordination. Without competition, there will be no progress in science. The essence of competition in science is to "compete" by enhancing one's own strength, and the core of cooperation for progress is to "cooperate" with the vision of mutual benefits, both of which aim at improving oneself to represent the world-level science and technology and to lead advance in science and technology. Scientists need to share ideas with each other. Coordination is required when they reserve different opinions since only teamwork can achieve "big" science.

Infectious diseases know no borders. A typical case is when "ambulances run through the streets of Toronto, Canada after a sneeze in Hong Kong, China." In this case, an infected Hong Kongese sneezed and passed the virus on to an elderly tourist from Toronto during the outbreak of SARS. After the elderly tourist returned home by air, many people in Toronto contracted "SARS," leading to frequent calls for ambulance services. Someone may think he is far away from these infectious diseases. In fact, we are all just a plane ride away from exposure to any emerging infectious disease.

It is not alarmist to say that we are on the brink of a global crisis of infectious diseases. No country can be free from the potential destruction of this crisis, neither can they rest without worrying about it. People worldwide should be alert regarding global public security risks since novel pathogens are always mutating and will seize the opportunity to break out, spread, and threaten human health upon finding the loophole or weakness in the prevention system.

International cooperation in global health must be devoted to establishing a strong and sustainable disease control system, building professional and dedicated disease control teams, improving timely and accurate communication mechanisms, and developing a partnership network of interconnectivity and cooperation. While strengthening their own public health capacity, countries must assist other countries in improving their public health systems, like building prevention and control institutions in Africa. Only by building a sounder global health safety network based on mutual benefit and win-win results can we prevent all kinds of threats to health, usher in healthy and bright prospects for the well-being of people around the world, and perform a chorus of dreams in a new era on the international stage.

"The wise delight in water while the good delight in mountains. The wise love mobility while the good love tranquility. The wise live happy while the good live long" (*The Analects of Confucius*). The two stones in the Olympic Village campus of CAS, from countries involved in international cooperation, shared their happiness in witnessing green sea and blue sky, which are the testimony to the purpose of disease prevention and control and longevity.

Science Popularization refers to popularizing scientific and technological knowledge to the public, advocating scientific methods, transmitting scientific thoughts, and carrying forward the scientific spirit in an easy-to-understand way. Popular science contributes to public's understanding of health and hygiene, improves their awareness of disease prevention and control, and draws their attention to scientific knowledge and achievements. Science Popularization aims to jointly create and share a natural and social "big ecology" close to the public and enable them to have interest in science by means of activities and platforms, which integrate scientific knowledge with people's life for their involvement and exchanges.

In the exploration and discovery of innovative scientific and technological knowledge, scientists also shoulder the responsibility of telling science stories on the science and technology stage to the public. They are those with well balanced "good nature and accomplishments" who can facilitate both innovation and science popularization. Virus transmissions need no visa, nor does popular science. Advanced science and technology provides strong support to a powerful country, and the prosperous development of science and technology depends on the progress of carriers of science and technology.

Without the improvement of overall scientific quality of the public, it will be difficult to build up a large number of innovative and high-performance teams to rapidly translate scientific and technological achievements. The Olympic spirit "faster, higher, stronger" symbolizes that the most important thing is not winning but participating; the most important thing in life is not the triumph but the struggle; the essential thing is not to have conquered but to have fought well. Only when the science foundation is deeply rooted in the public psyche can they discover scientific brilliance by participation and achieve contentment through struggles.

Scientists should not only publish academic papers but also apply their scientific and technological achievements in promoting the great cause of modernization.

A century has passed since the 1918 pandemic struck the world. It seems that humans remain wandering in two diverged paths: one to death and war, and the other to health and peace. The path to health is a path with hardships and challenges, but also a path to extreme nobility and glory, a path to national rejuvenation, and even a path to a community with shared future for the whole world.

3. Community with Shared Future for Mankind

The year 2018 is destined to be a milestone in virology. The Global Virome Project will map the global spectrum of viruses to turn the unknown to the known and the passive into the active. The primate "host" will take actions this time.

The World Flu Day was established in 2018 in commemoration of the centenary of the devastating 1918 flu pandemic to arouse people's deeper understanding of influenza.

It is said in *The Art of War* by Sun Tzu, a Chinese military strategist, that "if you know your enemies and yourself, you can win a thousand battles without a single loss. If you only know yourself, but not you opponent, you may win or may lose. If you neither know yourself nor your enemy, you will always endanger yourself." Having a thorough knowledge of the situation of two sides, the army will be full of vigor without fatigue and exhaustion even after 100 battles. On the contrary, having no idea of the situation of both sides, the army will be extremely exhausted and lose its power once it starts fighting. The world's population grew from 1.6 billion to 6.9 billion from 1900 to 2010. Meanwhile, emerging infectious diseases caused by viruses never stopped spreading, with three novel viruses attacking humans almost every year.

Human's invasion and occupation of wildlife habitats accelerate the "spillover effect" of viruses from wildlife to humans, such as the variation and interspecies transmission of avian influenza viruses, the acute respiratory syndrome caused by coronavirus, the alarm over a high-risk pandemic raised by Ebola virus, and the next generations of humans threatened by Zika virus "flying out of the grass." Migratory birds, urban poultry, cave bats, desert camels, and rainforest mosquitoes are involved in these "epidemic wars." The viruses seem to have adapted to the given host's body. However, now, they have found a new host — humans.

People often fall into the trap of thinking where they "cannot see the wood for the trees." They draw a big circle and maybe go all the way across it, only to find that the virus is just one of the dots comprising a circle and it is themselves who draw this circle. We carry out assays on exploring the mysteries of viruses to fight viruses and viral diseases. However, we increase the risk of transmission of both natural and unnatural viruses, unintentionally or deliberately. From this perspective, it seems that it is time for us to think about exploring viruses "peacefully."

Today, it is known that there are about 1.5 million undiscovered viruses circulating in the wildlife. Now the majority of them can be discovered and analyzed, turning the limited unknown into the limited known, which enables humans to transform research on virology to big data research. Human response patterns will be converted by these information models to extend the limited known to the infinite unknown. The future of human health will be defended and protected through "proactive response" to the threat of the virus instead of the "past passive reaction."

By means of virus detection and sample collection, the Global Virome Project aims at obtaining big data on "viral ecology," including host range, geographical distribution, and epidemiology, meanwhile building a data library through viral genome sequencing in order to establish a super data viral spectrum integrating natural viral ecology and genetics. Based on the revolutionary upgrading model, the Global Virome Project will provide a public health "tool kit" for the world and a global database of viral threats and infectious diseases for new responses and initiatives to future threats.

In this Project, humans can compare and analyze thousands of members in each virus family and describe details of each virus's characteristics, its host ranges, geographical distribution, and epidemiology, so as to identify viruses with the most potential threats for adopting measures to prevent "spillover." In other words, the Project helps humans "win a hundred battles without a single loss" when fighting a certain virus type, rather than "always endanger themselves" every time in fighting a single virus.

As "virus pools" in nature, birds and mammals are the focus of the Project, which will cover 68.5% of the world's mammalian viruses to obtain 85% of the information about global virus groups, thereby greatly enriching our knowledge concerning viruses and life.

On February 23, 2018, *Science* published an article describing the Global Virome Project aimed to launch. On March 12, 2018, WHO released the list of potential disease threats. Diseases listed are those that may cause public health crises but lack effective drugs or vaccines. It is imperative to study these diseases as soon as possible. As expected, these viral diseases include Crimean–Congo hemorrhagic fever, Ebola, MERS, SARS, and Zika; surprisingly, a disease called "X" is also listed. Though the definition of disease "X" is extremely complex by WHO, it can be concluded as unknown diseases caused by unknown pathogens.

WHO sounds the alarm on prevention and preparation for disease "X" to the people worldwide maybe because WHO predicts that the Global Virome Project will lead to further invasion into wildlife territories that may bring unknown pathogens to human world or maybe because WHO foresees unknown novel pathogens will inevitably be discovered, or maybe because of both.

Reviewing the past century, influenza viruses have been with humans at almost every moment in human history, during which viruses came and went, and some of them returned. Since the end of the 20th century, three great projects in life science have been launched: the Human Genome Project, Human Microbiome Project, and the Global Virome Project.

The Human Genome Project has determined the nucleotide sequence of three billion base pairs in the DNA of the human genome, covering 99% of gene regions contained in the human genome with an accuracy of 99.99%. Humans are not the only organisms on earth. There are about 10 times as many microbes in the human body as there are human cells, and the number of microbial genomes is 100 times greater than that of our human genome. The Human Microbiome Project will study relationships of microorganisms to each other and to their hosts or environment. Mysteries of viruses and microorganisms, viruses and humans, and viruses and environment will be gradually discovered. However, when

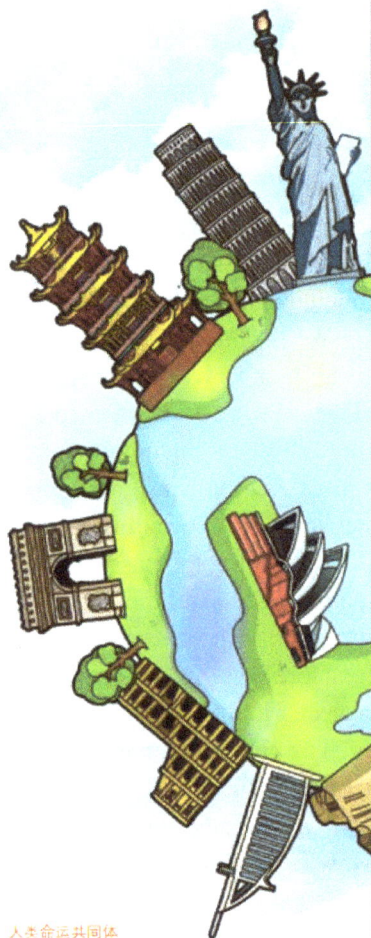

人类命运共同体

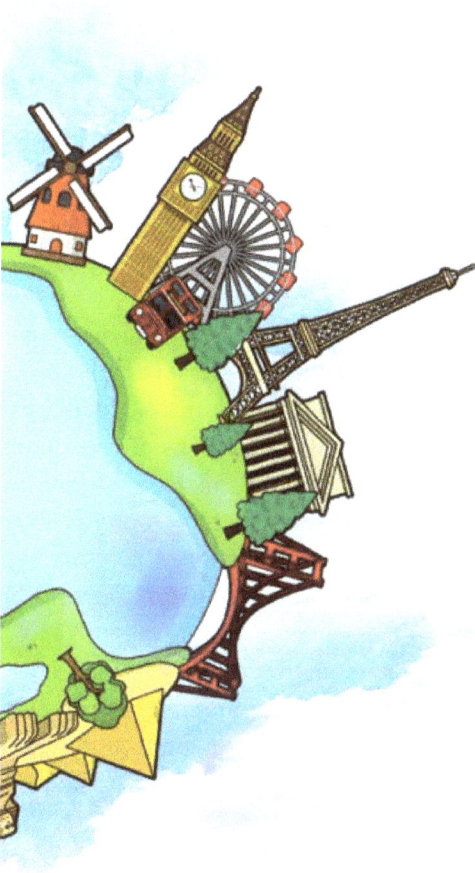

A Community with Shared Future for Mankind

reviewing the original mission of all projects, we will find that human beings are the core theme of all projects.

In the long history of the world, "round sky and square earth" is a basic concept in the tradition of ancient Chinese geography. The sky was like a dome with eight supporting props, while the earth was like a chessboard, which was converted into Jiuzhou (a poetic name for China) surrounded by oceans, giving birth to all living things. As in the poem *The Sea* written by Cao Cao, "The sun by day, the moon by night, Appear to rise up from the deep. The Milky Way with stars so bright, Sinks down into the sea in sleep." For a long time, the Western civilization regarded "geocentrism" as the core cosmology, and used the beautiful fairy tale to name the sun god, "Apollo," who orbited the Earth. It was not until the scientific discovery of "heliocentrism" that humans came to realize that the Earth was not the center of the Universe. Now we know that the sun is located in the Milky Way and the Milky Way is in the universe which was born with the Big Bang.

Viruses, which cannot even "stand on their own," threaten humans every now and then. Compared to humans, viruses are so simple in that they have only one goal: survival. Humans also need to survive, which can be achieved with concerted efforts of hundreds of millions of cells in our body and interactions of microbial cells in our body, including non-pathogenic viruses inhabiting cells. We are endowed with all resources on this blue planet and created the splendid human civilization. Have you ever seriously thought that all these endowments are gifts from the earth as well as love and care from nature?

Repeating wars and diseases throughout human history caused so many deaths. The air and water indispensable for our survival may enter into an irreversibly fragile state. The biodiversity and natural resources in the environment may no longer meet the bottom line of sustenance required for the ecological cycle.

In the past 100 years, humans stepped out of the shadows of the virus and explored the world of viruses to protect their health; forged ahead in the clinical practice and achieved one medical breakthrough after another with strong scientific and technological support; became stronger in the worldwide battle for disease control and built a community of shared future for mankind in the cause of global health. Humans overcame gravitational forces and tried to explore the universe beyond the biosphere and created the virtual spiritual home and oasis. Now it is time to return to reality to uphold world peace.

In the battle for the survival of the human race, influenza viruses are the enemies that are impossible to avoid.

One Hundred Years of the Flu Pandemic: The Milestone

1918	The "Spanish flu" pandemic
1931	Pathogen identification of swine influenza virus
1933	Pathogen identification of human influenza virus
1936	Chick embryo cultures of influenza virus
1940	Identification of influenza B virus
1941	HA/HAI assays based on agglutinate erythrocyte
1942	Neuraminidase (NA) activity identified
1945	Inactivated influenza vaccines licensed
1947	Establishment of the Global Influenza Programme and World Influenza Center by WHO
1950	Identification of influenza C virus
1957	Discovery of interferon
1957	H2N2 flu pandemic
1959	Negative stain viral structure obtained under an electron microscope
1966	Amantadine licensed for use against influenza A virus
1966	Cold-adapted viruses for use as live attenuated vaccines
1967	Antigenic association between human and animal influenza viruses recognized
1968	H3N2 flu pandemic
1969	Development of high-yielding reassortant vaccine viruses

1971	Protein composition characterization of influenza virus
1971	Human and animal reassortant viruses considered as the origin of pandemics
1975	Single radial diffusion assay was used as standard for vaccine potency
1976	Genome composition characterization of influenza virus
1977	Another human H1N1 influenza pandemic
1978–1982	All eight genome segments of influenza A virus sequenced
1979	Discovery of cap-dependent RNA transcription
1980	Integrated classification of subtypes of influenza A virus
1981	Hemagglutinin (HA) associates the pathogenicity of avian influenza virus
1981	The structure of HA antigen defined by monoclonal antibodies
1981	X-ray crystal structure of HA; the molecular mechanism of antigen mutation and receptor binding
1982	Changes in HA structure associated with membrane fusion at a low PH
1983	Identification of species differences in specific receptors of influenza A virus
1983	X-ray crystal structure of NA
1983	Genetic characteristics of Mx restriction factor gene
1985	M2 identified as target of amantadine
1986	The molecular mechanism of peptide recognition by T cells
1989	Reverse genetic manipulation of influenza viruses
1990	Establishment of PCR diagnosis and surveillance
1993	Structure-based design of NA inhibitor (Zanamivir)
1994	Identification of the polymerase promoter element
1996	M2 identified as a proton-selective channel
1997	First case of human infection with H5N1 in Hong Kong, China
1995–1998	NS1 inhibited interferon-mediated antiviral responses
1999	Zanamivir and Oseltamivir licensed for use against influenza A and B viruses
1999	Plasmid-based reverse genetic construction of influenza viruses

2003	The approval of live attenuated nasal spray vaccine
2005	Reconstruction of the 1918 pandemic virus
2006	Global Initiative on Sharing All Influenza Data (GISAID)
2008	Human broad-spectrum monoclonal antibodies as therapeutic candidates
2009	H1N1 flu pandemic
2011	WHO Pandemic Influenza Preparedness Framework ratified
2012	Approval of cell culture-derived influenza vaccine
2013	First case of human infection with H7N9 in China
2014	X-ray crystal structure of influenza polymerase trimer
2018	Approval of the first antiviral drug targeting the polymerase
2018	"World Flu Day" initiatives in Shenzhen, China

Recommended by Prestigious Experts

The current vaccine development and preparation are not able to keep up with the rapid mutations of various influenza viruses. But it is believed that humans will eventually hit the Achilles' heel by discovering the law of variations.

An excellent popular science book which tells China's story well and presents centenary influenza legends.

Qide Han (Member of the Chinese Academy of Sciences, Honorary President of China Association for Science and Technology, former Vice-Chairperson of the Standing Committee of the National People's Congress, and former Vice-Chairperson of the National Committee of the Chinese People's Political Consultative Conference)

Viruses know no national borders. The whole world is a community when fighting them. Reviewing the past century in fighting influenza viruses, we set off once again.

A centenary review of influenza viruses and a wonderful song to popularize science.

Zhu Chen (Member of the Chinese Academy of Sciences, the Vice-Chairperson of the Standing Committee of the National People's Congress, and President of Western Returned Scholars Association)

A healthy China is the call of the new era. Science is the core weapon and the public are the sources of strength in fighting against influenza viruses.

The book is both a centenary commemoration for the outbreak of the global pandemic and a glimpse of scientific and technological innovation in a new era.

Wei He (Professor at the Chinese Academy of Medical Sciences, Vice-Chairperson of the National Committee of the Chinese People's Political Consultative Conference, and Executive Vice-Chairperson of the Central Committee of the Agricultural and Labor Party)

It is everyone's responsibility to keep healthy and it is everyone's right to know influenza viruses and enjoy a healthy life.

Influenza viruses are talked about in the book by means of reviewing medical science in different civilizations in a science-popularized way to help readers know viruses and enjoy a healthy future.

Longde Wang (Member of the Chinese Academy of Engineering, President of Chinese Preventive Medicine Association, and "Healthy China 2020 Strategy Research Group" Chief Expert)

To know influenza viruses as well as prevent and control diseases is based on scientific and technological innovation for the cause of health.

The book brings a micro world of influenza viruses to readers to help them experience wonderful moments in infectious disease prevention and control, enjoy the innovative road to a healthy life, and witness the golden light of science and technology.

Yunde Hou (Member of the Chinese Academy of Engineering, winner of the State Preeminent Science and Technology Award, and Chief Technologist of the Special Major Science and Technology for Infectious Disease Prevention and Control)

To know influenza viruses, to explore life mysteries, and to spread science spirit.

The book integrates medicine into daily life and turns science and technology into art by putting thoughts into words and composing wonderful movements on health.

Chen Wang (Member of the Chinese Academy of Engineering, Vice-President of Chinese Academy of Engineering, President of Peking Union Medical College, Chinese Academy of Medical Sciences)

Are viruses really so scary? Influenza viruses come and go. Stay true to our mission and save lives.

The book helps readers to explore the knowledge valley and science ocean. It is a symphony of influenza and humans, diseases and health, as well as viruses and life.

Lanjuan Li (Member of the Chinese Academy of Engineering, Vice-President of Chinese Preventive Medicine Association, and Director of the Department of Biology and Medicine, Ministry of Education of the People's Republic of China)

An influenza pandemic occurred a century ago, and the small virus was found a century later. It is a silent battle lasting a century.

An exciting popular science book and an attractive literary work.

Yanhao Xu (Member of the Standing Committee of the National People's Congress, a member of the NPC Education, Science, Culture and Public Health Committee, and Vice President of China Association for Science and Technology)

Viruses have lived on the earth for at least three billion years like ghosts, and coexisted with humans for millions of years. It has not been a long time since we recognized them, but our scientific cognition will become the ultimate weapon to defeat them.

The book is a treasury of knowledge on the eternal topic of health. The heartrending stories in it release the discoveries that have changed our destiny.

Zhonghe Zhou (Member of the Chinese Academy of Sciences, Chairman of the International Paleontological Society, and Chairman of the China Science Writers Association)

Glossary of Terms and Definitions

A

Acquired Immune Deficiency Syndrome (AIDS) is a major infectious disease caused by HIV infection. The virus mainly attacks and destroys the immune system, making people susceptible to many diseases and generate malignant tumors.

Active Immunity is the process of exposing the individual to a live pathogen or of vaccination to generate a strong adaptive immune response to the subsequent infections. Passive immunity is the specific immunity that the body obtained by passively receiving antibodies and sensitized lymphocytes or their products. Passive immunity provides immediate but short-lived protection, such as diphtheria antitoxin.

Acute Respiratory Distress Syndrome (ARDS) is characterized by acute onset, difficulty in breathing, and hypoxemia, which is difficult to be corrected by conventional oxygen therapy. With various causes and complex pathogenesis, ARDS is difficult to be identified and detected. The therapy mainly includes mechanical ventilation treatment and non-mechanical ventilation treatment.

Adjuvant is the substance that can change or improve the specific immune response in the body to antigens and performs auxiliary functions. Adjuvants can induce the body to produce longer-lasting and highly-effective specific immune response to protect itself, thus minimizing the dose of antigen needed to cut the cost of developing vaccines. At present, there are different classes of adjuvants based on their chemical compositions, including aluminum salt adjuvants, protein adjuvants, nucleic acid adjuvants, lipid adjuvants, and mixed adjuvants.

American Plague occurred during the Europeans' Great Navigations period. There were only indigenous people living in the Americas at the arrival of European explorers. As European explorers expanded their activities there, they had conflicts and wars with the indigenous people, leading to the spreading of diseases in the New World, especially highly infectious diseases such as smallpox. The indigenous people lacked immunity to these diseases, resulting in widespread diseases and death, which exerted an important influence on civilization and history of the Americas.

Amoeba, living in water, soil, or decaying organic matter, is distributed worldwide. It is often regarded to be unrelated to human diseases. As a host of giant viruses such as Pandoravirus, amoeba can provide animal model systems for research.

Anthrax is an acute zoonotic infectious disease caused by *Bacillus anthracis*. Under natural conditions, herbivores such as cattle, horses, sheep, and camels are main sources of anthrax infections in humans, who will be infected through contact with infected animals or contaminated animal products or their meat. Main clinical symptoms include skin necrosis, ulceration, eschar and extensive edema of surrounding tissues, and toxemia, which result in acute infections in lungs, intestines, and meninges with sepsis complication. Severe symptoms can even lead to death.

Antitoxic Serum is a serum resisting a specific toxin or attenuating even inactivating the virulence. It is prepared by repeatedly injecting small quantities of the toxin produced by snake venom and pathogenic bacteria into the blood vessels of rabbits and horses. After a certain period, the antitoxin will be produced in the animal body. The antitoxin is then separated from the blood and purified for making antitoxic serum.

Archaea are members of the third branch of life in the tree of life using rRNA sequence. The other two common branches are Bacteria and Eukarya. Living in extreme environments, such as hot springs, anoxic lakes, and saline lakes, Archaea possess unique biochemical properties, thereby becoming a special life form.

Athens Plague occurred in 430 B.C. and nearly destroyed civilized Athens at that time. The historian Thucydides, who was present and contracted the disease himself and survived, described the epidemic: healthy young people suffer from a sudden fever, hyperemia of throat and tongue, extremely foul-smelling breath, and coughing and chest pain. People used fire to prevent the plague and avoid the ensuing disaster, while Athens citizens lived in fear and developed nightmares about the disease.

B

Basophil contains basophilic granules in cells and is found in a very small number in the blood. Granules consist of histamine, heparin, and allergic slow reacting substances, which have the function of anticoagulation, capillary permeability regulation, and smooth muscle contraction, and are associated with allergic reactions in the body.

B/SEAL/Netherlands/1/99 is the standard method for naming influenza viruses in terms of subtype/host/isolation country/number/collection date, i.e., Influenza B virus/SEAL/Netherlands/No.1/1999.

B Lymphocytes, also known as B cells, originate from stem cells in the bone marrow, which gradually differentiate into B cells after moving to the bursa of Fabricius or cystic organs. Mainly distributed in lymph nodes and spleen, B cells mainly play a role in humoral immune response by differentiating into plasma cells to produce antibodies with the stimulation of antigens.

Broth Experiment is the swan-neck flask experiment designed by Pasteur. He poured the broth into two flasks, the first with the upright neck and the second with the swan neck. The broth was boiled and cooled in two open flasks to expose the broth to the air. He left the two flasks in the lab for three days and found that the broth in the first flask became cloudy indicating microbial contamination, while second flask was sterile. Several months, or even a year later, the second flask remained clear without microbial contamination. It turned out that there was no spontaneous generation and microorganisms in the air were responsible for the deterioration of the broth since it was the microorganism that gave birth to new microbial lives.

C

Carbolic Acid, also known as Phenol, is a chemical compound with a specific odor found in coal tar. It is a key ingredient for bactericides, preservatives, and drugs (like aspirin) and can be used directly as the preservative and disinfectant solution.

Cervical Cancer, with HPV as a common pathogen, is a cervical tumor, the most common malignant tumor developed in women. The incidence of cervical cancer is not the same in different regions.

Chikungunya Virus (CHIKV), mainly transmitted by *Aedes albopictus* and *Aedes aegypti*, can cause Chikungunya with clinical symptoms similar to those of Dengue fever. The person infected with Chikungunya virus develops such typical symptoms as muscle pains, and even fever, nausea, and vomiting in severe cases, which may be complicated by meningitis. It frequently occurs in tropical Africa and Asia.

Chromosome, a special form of genetic material in a cell, mainly consists of DNA and proteins. It is species-specific and varies in number, size, and shape in different species, cell types, and development stages. In humans, each cell normally contains 23 pairs of chromosomes, for a total of 46. Twenty-two of these pairs, called autosomes, look the same in both males and females. The 23rd pair, the sex chromosomes, consists of two

X chromosomes in most females, and an X chromosome and a Y chromosome in most males.

Clone, with Chinese transliteration "Ke Long," refers to the population of any organism whose genetic information is identical to that of a parent organism by asexual reproduction in somatic cells. It can also be regarded as using biotechnology to asexually produce the individual or population with identical genes to those of their parents.

Conserved Sequence is a nucleotide fragment or an amino acid fragment of a protein in the DNA molecule that remains relatively unchanged. The conserved sequences are highly identical or similar in different molecules across species or in the same organism.

Cowpox, caused by vaccinia virus, is an acute infectious disease of cattle. Vaccinia virus has antigenic properties similar to the smallpox virus that causes human smallpox. Local ulcers usually occur in the udder of a cow and can be transmitted to humans via contact, with milkers and slaughterhouse workers as the susceptible population. Infected patients will develop skin rash, blisters, pustules, and other mild symptoms.

Crystallization is a chemical process where crystals precipitate from the solute when the host saturated solution cools. The crystal, which is usually made of a pure substance, is the solid formed by atoms, ions, or molecules arranged in a spatial ordered structure.

Cytokine (CK) is low-molecular-weight protein that is synthesized and secreted by the stimulation of immune or non-immune cells. With various biological activities, cytokines have a wide array of functions such as regulating cell growth, differentiation and effect, modulating immune responses and cell growth, and repairing damaged tissues, by means of binding to corresponding receptors such as interleukins, interferon, and growth factors.

Cytotoxic T Lymphocyte (CTL), also known as killer T cell, is the cell that monitors and kills target cells when necessary. The immune system detects target cells with specific antigens to stimulate the generation of effector cytotoxic T cells that can eliminate infected cells or cancer cells.

D

Dendritic Cells (DCs) are named for their probing tree-like shapes at the stage of maturation. With strongest functions, Antigen Presenting Cells (APCs) can efficiently ingest, process and present antigens and activate initial T cells. They play a central role in the initiation, regulation and maintenance of immune responses.

Dengue Virus (DENV), which is mainly transmitted by the bite of insect vectors such as *Aedes aegypti* and *Aedes albopictus* infected with a dengue virus, causes Dengue fever and Dengue shock syndrome. As an epidemic in tropical and subtropical areas, it is a widespread viral infectious disease with a high incidence rate.

Diffuse Alveolar Damage (DAD) is a pathologically descriptive term in association with clinical symptoms such as difficulty breathing and diffuse pulmonary infiltrates.

Diphtheria is an acute respiratory infectious disease caused by strains of bacteria called *Corynebacterium diphtheriae* that generate toxins. It can lead to fever, difficulty in breathing, hoarseness, barking cough, and white pseudomembrane developing over pharynx, palatine tonsils and surrounding tissues. In severe cases, systemic poisoning symptoms are obvious with complications of myocarditis and peripheral nerve paralysis. It is mainly transmitted via respiratory droplets.

Disulfide Bond (S–S) is a chemical bond formed by sulfur-containing amino acids linking different peptide chains or different parts of the same peptide chain. As a relatively stable covalent bond, it plays a role in stabilizing the spatial structure of the peptide chain of protein molecules. In general, more disulfide bonds mean greater stability of protein molecule against external factors.

DPT vaccine is short for Diphtheria–Pertussis–Tetanus vaccine. The vaccine, which is composed of pertussis vaccine, refined diphtheria, and tetanus toxoids in appropriate proportion, protects against diphtheria, pertussis, and tetanus.

E

Electron Diffraction Experiment refers to when a wave bypasses an obstacle and continues to transmit, which is called wave diffraction in classic physics. Electron diffraction experiments on crystals were found when electrons were accelerated by an electric field with wavelengths below the size of atoms. It is applied in the development of electron microscopy.

Emerging and Re-emerging Infectious Diseases (EID) is a concept proposed according to the discovery time of diseases. Emerging infectious diseases are those caused by new pathogens or pathogenic strains, such as MERS and influenza, and re-emerging infectious diseases are those caused by the reappearance of known pathogens like rabies and Ebola.

Endocytosis is a cellular process in which substances are brought into the cell. The biomacromolecules and particle substances attached to the cell membrane are internalized and surrounded by an area of cell membrane, which then buds off inside the cell to form a vesicle containing ingested substances.

Epidemiology is the study of diseases, health conditions, distribution, and their determinants in defined populations, as well as strategies and measures for disease prevention and health promotion.

Epidemic Encephalitis B (EEB) is caused by the Japanese Encephalitis Virus (JEV). It was discovered in Japan and thus was also known as Japanese Encephalitis B. It is a mosquito-borne blood infectious disease mainly distributed in the Far East Asia and Southeast Asia. Clinical symptoms at acute onset include fever, impaired consciousness, spasms, and meningeal stimulation. Severe symptoms often leave sequelae, leading to respiratory or circulatory failure and death.

Epithelial Cell is the cell that lines the surface of the skin or cavities. It is flat or columnar and mainly found on the nasal cavity, nasopharynx, organs, lungs, stomach, intestines, and other organs. Epithelial cells are different in organs. For example, functions of epithelial cells on cavities include secretion, excretion, and absorption; the outer layer of the skin is composed of keratinized epithelial cells with protective and absorptive functions.

Epitope, the chemical group on the antigen surface, determines the specific structures of the antigen, which is capable of stimulating an immune response by activating lymphocytes through binding antigens and corresponding lymphocyte surface antigen receptors. An antigen molecule has one or more different epitopes, while an epitope has only one antigen specificity, which is the basis of specific immune response.

Etiology is the study of causes of diseases.

Ebola Virus (EBOV), the pathogen to hemorrhagic fever, is a filamentous particle mainly transmitted through the blood, saliva, sweat, and secretions of the patients to cause intestinal, non-gastrointestinal, or intranasal infections. A variety of non-human primates are generally susceptible to it. As the deadliest infectious disease, Ebola hemorrhagic fever can kill the infected people within a short period of time after disease onset.

Escherichia coli (*E. coli*) is a type of bacteria that normally lives in your intestines causing extra-intestinal infections. Most types of *E. coli* are harmless. But some strains, generally called pathogenic *E. coli*, are highly pathogenic, meaning they can cause diarrhea as well as other diseases.

F

Ferret, whose wild habitat is the forest and semi-forest near water sources, can be domesticated and is sensitive to human influenza virus.

Infected ferrets have similar symptoms to that exhibited by humans. Therefore, they are important animal models for the human influenza virus.

Formaldehyde, also named methanal, dissolves easily in water and ethanol. The 37% aqueous solution is usually called formalin. Formaldehyde is a colorless liquid with a strong pungent odor and reducing property. With protein denaturation and antiseptic and bactericidal properties, it can be used to soak biological specimens and biological products.

G

Gas Weapon, the man-made chemical weapon for military purposes, is a general term for gases harmful to living organisms. Gas weapons such as chlorine gas caused heavy casualties on both sides in battlefields of World War I.

Gene, a functional nucleic acid sequence, is a carrier of life functions and information. It was found in the Human Genome Project that humans have far fewer genes than previously thought and the protein genetic sequence produced makes up 1.5% of the total DNA length.

Glycoprotein is the protein containing oligosaccharide chains covalently attached to amino acid side-chains, with the biological function of biometric identification of cells or molecules.

Guillain–Barré Syndrome (GBS) is an autoimmune peripheral neuropathy characterized by demyelination of peripheral nerves and nerve roots and small blood vessel inflammatory cells infiltration, with clinical symptoms of symmetric acute flaccid paralysis.

H

Hemorrhagic Fever is a serious infectious disease caused by epidemic hemorrhagic fever viruses. It is mainly transmitted via mucosa or damaged skin with symptoms such as fever, bleeding tendency, and visceral damage. As an acute viral infectious disease, it is widespread with a high fatality rate.

Hepatitis B is an infectious disease caused by Hepatitis B Virus (HBV). People are infected via blood, sex, or mother-to-child transmission. Patients with chronic conditions may develop liver cirrhosis, and a few may develop liver cancer.

Human Immunodeficiency Virus (HIV) is the pathogen to Acquired Immune Deficiency Syndrome. It is roughly spherical. Its viral envelope proteins consists of glycoprotein (gp) 120 and gp41, which mainly target CD4 T lymphocytes in the human immune system. It destroys large numbers of CD4 T lymphocytes, resulting in immunodeficiency in the body. Therefore, it is known as Human Immunodeficiency Virus.

Hydrogen Bond is a special intermolecular or intramolecular force when Hydrogen atoms bind to same or different atoms, such as hydrogen bonds between H_2O and H_2O, or NH_3 and H_2O.

I

ICU (Intensive Care Unit), also known as the intensive therapy unit, is a special department that caters to patients with severe or life-threatening illnesses and injuries, which require constant care, close supervision from life support equipment, advanced technology, and medication in order to ensure normal bodily functions.

Interferon (IFN) is a highly species-specific glycoprotein which was first discovered in the cell membrane of a chick embryo. Interferon was named for its ability to "interfere" with influenza virus infection. It is a family of multifunctional cytokines with broad-spectrum antiviral, antiproliferative, and immunomodulatory activities.

Intestinal Flora is the microorganism living in the digestive tracts of humans. For example, *Bifidobacterium* and *Lactobacillus* play significant roles in human health by affecting immune response to infections through synthesizing a variety of vitamins and amino acids required for the growth and development of the body, involving in carbohydrate and protein metabolism, and helping the body to absorb such microelements as iron and zinc.

Ion Transporter is the transmembrane protein that moves ions across membrane and maintains their concentration at a normal level in different cell compartments. As a type of membrane protein, ion transporter mediates chemical substances and signal exchanges inside and outside biological membranes and plays an important role in cell activities such as nutrient uptake, metabolite releases, and signal transduction.

L

Lipid Bilayer, the basic scaffold of cell membrane, is a mobile biomembrane. Phospholipid, which accounts for 50%–60% of lipid bilayer, is a molecule composed of glycerol, fatty acid, and phosphoric acid. The phosphoric acid has a hydrophilic head and the fatty acid has a hydrophobic tail. The two layers of phospholipid bind their "tails" to provide an isolated environment for cells. Most phospholipid and protein molecules that make up cell membranes are able to move. Some protein molecules are bound to the surface of the lipid bilayer, some are partially or completely embedded in lipid bilayer, and others can cross the lipid bilayer. Featured by selective permeability, cell membranes can proceed life activities in order.

Lymph Nodes/Trimer are oval or bean-shaped lymphoid tissues surrounded by blood vessels. Lymph nodes are concentrated in concealed concaves in the body, such as axilla, groin, organ hilum, or near great vessels of the chest and abdomen. There are hundreds of lymph nodes throughout the body. Some are deep inside the body, and some are shallow. Lymph nodes can produce lymphocytes and antibodies to remove bacteria and foreign substances.

Lysozyme is an alkaline enzyme that hydrolyzes mucopolysaccharides in pathogenic bacteria. It dissolves insoluble mucopolysaccharides cell walls into soluble sugar peptide and causes cell walls rupture and content escape to dissolve bacteria. Lysozyme has antibacterial and anti-inflammatory effects.

M

Mast cell, the tissue cell with strong basophilic particles, is widely distributed around microvessels under the skin and visceral mucosa. It secrets a variety of cytokines involved in regulating immune response, expresses large numbers of immunoglobulin E receptors, and releases allergic mediators with weak phagocytic functions.

Measles Virus (MV), the pathogen to Measles, is highly contagious. Classic signs of measles include skin rash, fever, and respiratory symptoms. It is transmitted via droplets or close contact with utensils and toys. With a high incidence rate to the susceptible, it is a common acute infectious disease in children.

Microbes are tiny living organisms that are found all around us, including fungi, bacteria, viruses, etc.

Middle East Respiratory Syndrome Coronavirus (MERS-CoV) is the MERS pathogen. It was first discovered in Saudi Arabia and was prevalent in the Middle East. It is the sixth known human coronavirus, with clinical symptoms of fever, chills, cough, shortness of breath, muscle pain, and even acute respiratory distress syndrome.

Miller's Experiment is a chemical experiment that simulates the reductive atmosphere thought to be present on the early earth to generate organic substances in simulated thunders and lightning and tests the chemical origin of life under those conditions. It was conducted in 1953 by Stanley Miller, with assistance from Harold Urey, at the University of Chicago. The experiment used CH_4, NH_3, and H_2 to simulate the reducing atmosphere, which was then mixed with H_2O. After a week of continuous operation of simulated thunder and lightning, 20 organic substances were yielded, including 11 amino acids. Four yielded amino acids were present in biological proteins, which proved the atmosphere on the early earth may turn inorganic substance into low molecular weight organic ones.

Molecular Evolution is the evolution of biological macromolecules in the process of biological development. Changes and evolutionary relationships of biological molecules can be analyzed and calculated by using molecular biology data to construct phylogenetic trees of biological groups.

Monoclonal Antibody (mAb) is the antibody made by a single B-cell clone to target a specific antigen epitope. Hybridoma technology is usually used for preparation, in which mouse myeloma cells cultured in vitro and proliferated in large quantities are fused with pure mouse B cells secreted by antigen immunization to form hybrid cell lines, which can be used to prepare the specific antibody against an antigen epitope, namely the monoclonal antibody.

Mouse refers to the white fur laboratory mouse widely used in medicine, pharmacy, biology, and other teaching and research activities. There are many mouse varieties after long-term selection and directional breeding, which can be generally divided into common mice and special mice for specific demand.

mRNA (Messenger RNA) is a single-stranded RNA molecule transcribed by the DNA template. mRNA is then used as the template where proteins are made. In addition to mRNA, there are tRNA, rRNA, and miRNAs playing the roles of transport, assembly, and regulation in the life process, respectively.

Mumps Virus (MV), the pathogen to Mumps, can cause swelling parotid gland, sublingual gland, submaxillary gland, headache, fever, and various complications. It is transmitted via droplet or contact. School-age children are susceptible to Mumps virus, which is more common in the winter and spring.

***Mycobacterium tuberculosis* (*M. tuberculosis*)**, also known as Tubercle Bacilli (TB), is the pathogen of tuberculosis (TB), which can cause inflammation in tissues and organs after massive replication. As a major infectious disease, the virulence of its bacterial compositions and metabolites causes damage to the body. Variations in virulence and drug resistance may occur. The bacteria can attack any part of the body, while TB of the lungs is the most common disease form.

N

Nipah Virus (NiV) is the pathogen to Nipah virus infection, a zoonotic disease. It was named after Nipah, the Malaysian village where it was first discovered. Its hosts include humans, pigs, as well as bats, and birds may help to spread the virus. It mainly affects the central nervous system and respiratory system, with clinical symptoms of encephalitis or respiratory disease. It can be transmitted via contact and has a high fatality rate.

Non-covalent Bond is a type of chemical bond that is different from a covalent bond. A covalent bond occurs when two or more atoms share the outermost layers of electrons to form relatively stable chemical structures by reaching electron saturation in ideal circumstances. A non-covalent interaction differs from a covalent bond in that it does not involve the sharing of electrons, but rather involves more dispersed variations of electro-magnetic interactions between molecules or within a molecule, such as ionic bonds and intermolecular forces.

O

Outbreak is a sudden appearance of something (a disease, especially an epidemic), which is different from the term "breakout." The latter also refers to a sudden appearance, but used in a wider extent, such as war or conflict breakout.

Ovalbumin is a phosphorous-containing glycoprotein found in egg white, making up approximately 54%–69% of the total protein in egg white. In the production and preparation of vaccines and biological drugs, ovalbumin is often used as a protein additive to improve their stability. Ovalbumin in egg white is the allergen in eggs, quail eggs, and other egg products.

P

Pandoravirus is a genus of giant virus with one micron in diameter. It is speculated that the virus may be originated in ancient times or even from other planets. Thus, scientists named it "Pandora."

Pathology is the study of causes, mechanisms, and development of human diseases as well as the morphological structure, functional metabolism, and pathological changes of the body during the course of diseases.

Pathogen is the microorganism that causes diseases, such as viruses, bacteria, and plasmodia.

Perforin is a glycoprotein found in body's immune cells such as lymphocytes. After close contact and interactions with target cells, perforin will be released and polyperforin tubular channels will be formed on target cell membranes, leading to the lysis and destruction of target cells.

Pestis is a highly infectious disease transmitted by rat flea infected with *Yersinia pestis*. It is widely prevalent in wild rodents. Clinical symptoms include fever, severe toxemia symptoms, swollen lymph nodes, pneumonia, and bleeding tendency. Pestis is a highly fatal disease that has caused plague outbreaks and pandemics throughout the world history.

pH is the ratio of the total number of hydrogen ions in the solution to the total number of substances. It can be determined by using pH indicators, pH dipsticks, or pH meters. At 25°C, solutions with a pH less than 7 are acidic, solutions with a pH greater than 7 are basic, and solutions with a pH equal to 7 are neutral.

Phage Display Technology is a biological technique that inserts a foreign protein or polypeptide DNA sequence into a phage coat protein gene, generating the foreign gene with the expression of coat protein and displaying the foreign protein on the surface of phage as it reassembles.

Phagocytin is an alkaline protein with bactericidal activity found in neutrophilic leukocytes.

Phosphodiester Bond occurs when two of the hydroxyl groups in phosphoric acid react with hydroxyl groups on another molecule to form two ester bonds, which become the bridge between two hydroxyls and forms polynucleotide chain, namely the nucleic acid macromolecule chain. The high stability of the phosphodiester bond is regarded as one of the key reasons for nucleic acids acting as genetic materials.

Plasma is the extracellular matrix of blood. It is a pale-yellow liquid consisting of proteins, lipids, inorganic salts, sugars, amino acids, metabolic wastes, and large amounts of water. It plays a vital role in transporting blood cells and materials essential to maintain human activities.

Point Mutation refers to alterations of a single base pairs, including replacement, insertion, or deletion. Point mutation generally has a high recovery mutation rate.

Poliomyelitis is an acute infectious disease caused by Poliovirus (PV) causing severe damage to children's health. It mainly infects motor nerve cells in the central nervous system, leading to flaccid paralysis in limbs, particularly in children. Thus, it is also named infantile paralysis.

Protein Conserved Region, with important genetic or physiological functions, is the similar region comprising different amino acid sequences of proteins or nucleotide sequences of different genes.

Plague/Pestilence is an infectious disease caused by highly pathogenic microorganisms, such as bacteria, and viruses.

Pre-natural Infection is the specific immunity that a person will develop if he is pre-infected with the virus. When he is inoculated the viral vector vaccine, it will be identified and eliminated by the immune system in the body, making the immune defense ineffective or weakened, which is an obstacle and challenge for vaccine design.

Provirus is the cDNA formed by reverse transcription of retrovirus RNA. Viral genomes are replicated and transcribed through a DNA intermediate, which is called provirus. Provirus can be integrated into the genome of a host cell and passed from an integrated parent host cell to a daughter host cell.

Pure Culture is the offspring reproduced from a cell or a group of identical cells culture in microbiology. A pure culture may originate from bacteria, viruses, and other microorganisms. Pure culture samples are generally required for identification.

R

Rabies is an acute infectious disease caused by the rabies virus, which usually infects dogs, wolves, and cats. Humans bit by infected animals have clinical symptoms as hydrophobia, ancraophobia, pharyngeal spasm, and progressive paralysis. Thus, it is also known as Hydrophobia. When a person is bitten by an infected animal, the virus in its saliva will enter the wound and cause disease. Human rabies is nearly 100% fatal since there remain few effective treatment approaches to it.

Rabies Virus (RV), the pathogen to rabies, is the rhabdovirus. Wild animals such as foxes, wolves, and bats are natural hosts of rabies. In human dwelling areas, dogs and cats are main infectious sources for rabies infections in human and domestic animals. It is widespread all over the world.

Reassortment is the switching of strong homologous gene segments in cells infected with different influenza viruses that have viral gene segments. Recombination is a process by which pieces of DNA are broken and recombined to produce new combinations of genes.

Resolution refers to the quality of an image, which determines the precision of image details. Image pixels consist of points, lines, and faces. In general, the higher the image resolution is, the more pixels the image contains, and the clearer the image.

Respiratory Tract, the passage through which air flows during lung breathing, is divided into upper airways and lower airways. Upper airways include nose, pharynx, and larynx. Lower airways include trachea, bronchi, and lung organs.

Reye Syndrome is a rare disease that occurs in children who have had a recent influenza infection. The cause of the disease remains unknown. It can result in rapid worsening liver and brain, and even death. It is necessary to give symptomatic and supportive clinical treatment in time.

Ribonucleic Acid (RNA), the genetic information carrier in cells and some viruses, is a linear molecule with ribose nucleotide attached to phosphodiester bonds. A ribonucleotide molecule consists of a phosphate group, a sugar ribose, and a nitrogenous base.

Rift Valley Fever Virus (RVFV), the pathogen of Rift Valley Fever, was first discovered and isolated in sheep in the Rift Valley of Kenya. It is mainly spread by the bite of infected mosquitoes or touching infected animals. The infected people can develop an acute zoonotic infectious disease with mild clinical symptoms such as fever and muscle pain. Severe symptoms may include bleeding, shock, encephalitis or hepatitis, and even death. Patients exhibiting bleeding symptoms have high chances of death.

Rodent has a single pair of incisors in each of upper and lower jaws. About 40% of all mammal species are rodents, such as rabbits and rats. They are the most diversified mammalian order and the most widely distributed mammal species in the world (around 2,000 species).

S

Salmonella typhi (*S. typhi*) is the pathogen to typhoid (different from cold damage disorders and the miscellaneous illness in traditional Chinese medicine). Strong release of endotoxin occurs when it is lysed, which will affect the intestinal lymphoid tissue, liver, spleen, as well as bone marrow and cause septicemia and organ damage. The infection is often passed on through contaminated water or contact with the person infected with typhoid.

Self-assembly is a technique in which basic substance units spontaneously form ordered structures. It occurs in molecules and in nanometer-, micron-, or larger-scale materials, and is usually organized or aggregated into a stable structure with a geometric appearance.

Septic Shock is a shock caused by sepsis, also known as infection throughout the body. Most cases of septic shock are caused by Gram-positive bacteria and mainly occurs in acute obstructive suppurative cholangitis, gangrenous cholecystitis, pyelonephritis, acute pancreatitis, and infectious diseases.

Severe Acute Respiratory Syndrome Coronavirus (SARS-CoV) is the pathogen causing Severe Acute Respiratory Syndrome, also known as SARS virus. Clinical symptoms include systemic symptoms such as fever, fatigue, headache, muscle and joint pain and respiratory signs such as dry cough, chest tightness, and difficulty breathing. Patients suffer obvious dyspnea in severe cases and can rapidly develop the acute respiratory distress syndrome.

Sick Cattle and Sheep refer to animals that died of infectious animal diseases, like anthracnose caused by *Bacillus anthracis*, which may infect humans. Sick and dead animals as well as contaminated soil, grassland, water, and feed are primary infection sources that lead to human infection and death.

Standard Curve is the curve representing values of properties by measuring physical and chemical properties of a series of existing components in a standard substance. Standard Curve is often used to establish a mathematical model of the functional relationship between physical or chemical properties of a standard substance and the instrument response.

Staphylococcus is named for its grape-like clusters. Most of Staphylococci are non-pathogenic bacteria widely distributed in nature. A few can cause diseases, including acute or chronic infectious diseases caused by *Staphylococcus aureus* infection.

T

Tetanus is a disease caused by an infection with the bacterium *Clostridium Tetani* in skin or mucosal wounds, which grows and reproduces in an anoxic environment in the body, generating toxins and muscle spasm. It is a specific trauma-associated infection.

T Lymphocytes, also known as T cells, originate from stem cells in the bone marrow. After developing to maturity in the thymus gland, they are distributed to immune organs and tissues over the body through lymphocytes and blood circulation. T cells play the central role in the immune response.

Tobacco Mosaic Disease is a plant infectious disease caused by the Tobacco Mosaic virus. The virus, mainly transmitted via sap, can invade the plant through large wounds or natural orifice, propagate in parenchyma cells, and enter vascular tissue to infect the whole plant. The virus can cause disease and even the death of plants at stages from seed to harvest, which is common in tobacco-growing areas around the world.

Transformation is the genetic and phenetic alteration of a cell resulting from the uptake and incorporation of exogenous genetic material from its surroundings. It is the earliest form of transferring genetic materials between bacteria.

Transmembrane Protein is the integral membrane protein that spans the lipid bilayer. The polypeptide chain of a transmembrane protein can span the membrane one or multiple time. The polypeptide chain is hydrophobic to span the hydrophobic region of the lipid bilayer and covalently bind to the fatty acid chain. The hydrophilic polar is located in the inner and outer surface of the membrane.

Tripolymer/Trimer is a product of polymer synthesis. It is a molecule polymerized by three identical molecules. There are some similar definitions like dimer, tetramer, pentamer, etc. They play corresponding biological functions.

V

Varicella is an acute contagious disease caused by the initial infection with Varicella-zoster Virus (VZV). The disease usually occurs in infants and preschool-age children, while is often more severe in adults than in children. It results in a characteristic skin rash, herpes, and scab. It is highly contagious and is mainly transmitted via respiratory droplets or direct contact.

Vibrio cholerae (***V. cholerae***), the pathogen of human cholera, produces enterotoxin, a severe diarrhea toxin, which affects the intestinal wall causing severe dehydration and collapse, and even metabolic acidosis and acute renal failure. Mainly transmitted through contaminated water or food via oral transmission, it has caused several pandemics in the world with clinical symptoms such as severe vomiting, diarrhea, dehydration, and high mortality rate.

Viremia is a medical condition where viruses enter the blood stream and hence have access to organs and central nervous system in the body, which may lead to organ failure or septicemia, and may even threaten life in severe cases.

W

Wave-particle Duality, one of the basic attributes of microscopic particles, is the concept that every particle or quantum entity may be described as either a particle or a wave.

X

X-ray is a particle beam produced by electron transitions from one energy level to another in an atom. It is the electromagnetic spectrum with the wavelength range between ultraviolet ray and gamma-ray. X-ray is also referred to as Röntgen radiation after the German scientist Wilhelm Röntgen, who discovered it. With the capacity of inducing different biological effects in vivo, X-ray radiation can be used in mutation breeding by inducing gene mutation in cells.

X-ray Diffraction Technology is the technique that uses the X-ray to diffract a crystal pattern on a photographic plate by radiating the crystal of substance. Periodic structures of the crystal enable it to produce the X-ray diffraction effect, through which reliable and accurate data about crystal structures can be obtained. With the data obtained, macromolecular structures and functions can be analyzed, such as proteins and DNA, which will be used for the design of molecular drug and research on structural function.

Y

Yellow Fever Virus (YFV), mainly transmitted by monkeys and other primates in tropical forests, is most contagious at early onset stages. Yellow fever virus invades the body and spreads to lymph nodes and replicates there. Several days later, it enters the bloodstream and generates a viremia. It usually occurs in Africa and South America.

Yersinia pestis (*Y. pestis*), the pathogen to pestis, causes bubonic plague, namely the Black Death. It generally infects rodents first and hops to humans through bites from infected rat fleas, which will be prevalent in the population via respiratory system.

Z

Zika Virus (ZIKV) is a member of the virus family Flaviviridae. It is an arbovirus transmitted by mosquitoes to wild primates and mosquito vectors such as Aedes mosquitoes. It becomes a public health emergency of international concern since the outbreak of Zika virus epidemic occurred in Brazil in 2015 and subsequent infections followed in many American and European countries.

Zoonosis is an infectious disease naturally transmitted between humans and livestock and poultry. It can be caused by pathogens such as viruses, bacteria, and protozoa and lead to diseases including rabies, influenza, mad cow disease, anthrax, tuberculosis, and schistosomiasis.

Postscript

First "World Flu Day" Advocated by China

The *Asian-Pacific Centenary Spanish 1918-flu Symposium* was held in Shenzhen, China, on November 1, 2018. China, in collaboration with relevant organizations at home and abroad, initiated the establishment of "World Flu Day" on November 1 to build up the world's confidence and determination in influenza prevention and control and to protect public health.

In 1918, the Spanish flu swept across the world and killed nearly 1 in 20 humans, making it the deadliest influenza pandemic in history. In 2018, reviewing the far-reaching havoc, leading experts on influenza virus from all over the world gathered for academic exchanges and collaboration on the influenza prevention and control in the Asia-Pacific region to prepare for a future influenza pandemic.

People remain helpless to deal with virus variations due to their limited knowledge about influenza despite the rapid development of science and technology worldwide. It is hoped that the symposium will inspire researchers, public health workers, and the public to attach great importance to influenza and will accelerate the development of innovative anti-influenza drugs and vaccines by strengthening basic and innovative research.

Experts present at the symposium from different countries shared their experience and reached consensus on influenza, a global health problem. Within the WHO coordination framework, a global influenza prevention and control system will be established to actively share information and promote international and regional cooperation. The future flu pandemic is inevitable, but we can work together to create a more protective world.

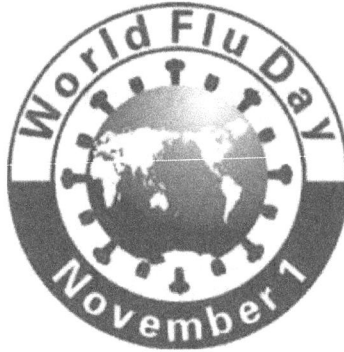

2018 年 11 月 1 日

November 1, 2018

Index

www.ingramcontent.com/pod-product-compliance
Lightning Source LLC
Chambersburg PA
CBHW050555190326
41458CB00007B/2046